The New
Honest Herbal

A Sensible Guide to the Use
of Herbs and Related Remedies

To Ginny, of course

THE NEW
HONEST HERBAL

A Sensible Guide to the Use
of Herbs and Related Remedies

Varro E. Tyler, Ph.D.

GEORGE F. STICKLEY COMPANY   210 W. WASHINGTON SQUARE
PHILADELPHIA, PA 19106

First Published 1982, The Honest Herbal
Second Edition, The New Honest Herbal

Copyright © 1987 by the George F. Stickley Company

Library of Congress Cataloging-in-Publication Data

Tyler, Varro E.
    The new honest herbal.

    Rev. ed. of: The honest herbal. 1981 or 1982.
    Bibliography: p.
    Includes index.
    1. Herbs—Therapeutic use.   2. Materia medica,
Vegetable.   I. Tyler, Varro E.   The honest herbal.
II. Title.
RM666.H33T94   1987   615'.321   87-9982
ISBN 0-89313-078-8

Printed and Manufactured in the United States and published by the George F. Stickley Company, 210 West Washington Square, Phila., Pa. 19106.

CONTENTS

vi

PREFACE

Medicine and quackery have always been close, if not compatible, partners. At times, they may appear to have separated, but sooner or later, in one place or another, they wind up reunited. The present area of greatest mutual attraction for them appears to be in the treatment of diseases by means of herbal remedies. More misinformation regarding the efficacy of herbs is currently being placed before consumers than at any previous time, including the turn-of-the-century heyday of patent medicines.

I had long wanted to write a popular herbal because, during three decades as a professional pharmacognosist, I had often wished to use this means to convey to others some of my interest in and enthusiasm for these fascinating natural drugs. But recently, after being exposed to some of the deluge of inaccurate and deceptive information which has appeared on the subject, I felt impelled to write about it. The result is this book.

The bulk of the useful information is contained in the write-ups on individual drugs which follow the introductory chapters. Most of them are organized according to a similar plan: a brief description of the drug and its proper nomenclature, as well as that of the plant from which it is derived, precede comments on its alleged uses. Then follows a nontechnical discussion of the chemistry and pharmacology (where known) of the active principles of the drug. Next is an evaluation based on all evidence known to the author which offers a judgment about the probable utility of the herb. Pertinent references to the literature conclude this discussion. These provide documentation for all significant statements and are possibly a unique feature of a book designed specifically for everyone interested in herbs. However, the references must be scrutinized carefully; some represent uncritical advocacy literature, others are scientific and authoritative. The context where each is cited will immediately clarify the type of literature involved.

Some readers will probably find fault with the information in this book, especially with the judgments presented. Some will find it too conservative, and it is, compared to the writings of most modern herbalists. Others may believe the volume is too liberal, promoting self-medication with self-selected herbs. That is a misconception. Self-medication is *not* being promoted. The information given only permits it to be done as intelligently as possible, if the reader wants to do so in the first place.

The lay reader, for the first time, is thus provided with accurate, scientific statements and reasoned judgments based on a recognized authority's lifetime of professional study of medicinal plants. Basic facts on the uses of herbs and related remedies are greatly needed, for interest in the entire field is tremendous and growing.

Because of this interest, it was impossible to cover all of the herbs of supposed medicinal value in a book of manageable size. One of the older listings of botanical drugs, J. M. Nickell's *Botanical Ready Reference*, first published a century ago, named 2526 different medicinal plants ranging from *Abelmoschus esculentus* (L.) Moench, the common okra, to *Zizia aurea* (L.) W.D.J. Koch, otherwise known as the meadow parsnip. The coverage could be extended even more if based on introductions since that time. Physical limitations aside, it is really not necessary to discuss all of these botanicals, for many are seldom encountered or are totally without value. The more than 100 included here were selected on the basis of relative significance to the public determined from literature sources (including retail and wholesale catalogs of herbs) and actual observation of products sold in "health food" stores.

There are three ways in which herbs are ordinarily obtained. The most common, in this era of urban living, is by purchase in a retail store. The problems in verifying the true identity of such products are discussed later. Some consumers may either choose to grow their own or to collect them from the wild. These options are completely beyond the scope of this book. While many recent herbal writings do encourage both activities, a word of warning is needed, especially in collecting wild plants. Make absolutely certain of the identity of the harvested material. Natural variations in different specimens can be misleading, and thus plant taxonomy (i.e., identification) is neither an exact science nor an easy one. Fatalities have been reported as a result of confusing and subsequently ingesting one wild plant for another.

Whether plant drugs are purchased or self-collected, it is important to remember that their active constituents may vary considerably, depending on: the conditions under which the plant was grown, the degree of maturity at the time of collection, the manner of drying, the conditions of storage, and other similar factors. These variables are overcome, in the case of crude drugs used in conventional medicine, by conducting chemical or physiological assays or tests and then standardizing the product by adding drug material of greater or lesser potency. The more potent the medicine, the more important it is that some sort of control be utilized to assure proper dosage. Unfortunately, herbs are seldom subjected to such procedures.

The information on the various herbs has been arranged in alphabetical order by common name for the convenience of the reader. Today, few people are able to place a particular plant in its proper family, let alone various families in their proper phylogenetic order. Imprecise as they are, common names have been used as titles simply because they are ones most people know. The imprecision in the system, I hope, has been overcome by comprehensive indexing.

Finally, remember as you read that your interest in herbs should be constructive, not destructive, to your health. This requires an ability not only to seek the truth but, after finding it, to discard any preconceived ideas which it may reveal as untrue.

> "Beware of the truth, gentle Sister. Although much sought after, truth can be dangerous to the seeker. Myths and reassuring lies are much easier to find and believe. If you find a truth, even a temporary one, it can demand that you make painful changes."

God Emperor of Dune
Copyright © 1981 by Frank Herbert
With permission of the author.

V.E.T.

West Lafayette, Indiana
December 1981

Preface to *The New Honest Herbal*

Much has happened in the field of herbal medicine since the manuscript for *The Honest Herbal* was completed more than five years ago. As predicted, some herbal enthusiasts found the information in that book too conservative. Consequently, many of the normal commercial outlets for such literature did not stock the book. It nevertheless received uniformly excellent critical acclaim from knowledgeable reviewers, and the original edition sold out completely.

In the interim, there have been some very encouraging developments in the field, stimulated I believe, in no small measure by *The Honest Herbal*. Several consumer-oriented groups, such as the National Council Against Health Fraud and the American Council on Science and Health, have begun to inform the public about the true utility of herbs. Several popular monthly newsletters, such as *Nutrition Forum* and *Tufts University Diet and Nutrition Letter*, have begun to feature articles disclosing the real facts about herbal products. It is significant to note, however, that these publications have as their primary focus the field of nutrition, not pharmacy or medicine. Many American journals and newsletters in these latter two areas still disdain authoritative articles dealing with herbs and their uses.

Consumer Reports, an extremely influential nationally circulated magazine devoted to examining product quality, has recently featured exposés of malpractice in the herbal field. And a very hopeful sign is the editorial reorientation of *Prevention*, a popular health magazine with 2.75 million circulation, toward a more conservative and genuinely helpful stance with regard to the utility of herbal products.

Events of this sort provided a considerable incentive to prepare a thorough revision of my original work. Consequently, the entire book has been revised and new material added, where appropriate, to produce *The New Honest Herbal*. It discusses encouraging new developments in the field of herbal regulation and control taking place in Canada. It contains new monographs on several important herbs, including butcher's-broom, capsicum, evening primrose, feverfew, ginger, pau d'arco, and schisandra. Some of the monographs, including those on aloe, hops, and yohimbine, contain important additions. All of the monographs have been carefully reviewed, and many are up-dated with significant new information and references.

The result is a volume of even greater significance than my

first effort to those interested in herbs. It is now made available in soft cover format so that it can reach a wider audience than its predecessor. I hope that all who read *The New Honest Herbal* will benefit from the uniquely honest and useful herbal information found within its pages.

V.E.T.

West Lafayette, Indiana
January 1, 1987

PROS AND CONS

The resurgence of interest in herbal medicine which originated during the last decade shows every promise of continuing its rapid development through the 1990's. Apparently, the movement had its origin in many people's disillusionment with modern medicine—its high cost and its inability to cure everything. This, along with the widespread belief that plant remedies were "naturally" superior to man-made drugs, produced a wave of enthusiasm and promotion on the part of the public which can only be described as an herbal renaissance.

Unfortunately, the partisans in the revival were more enthusiastic than knowledgeable, more evangelistic than critical. For reasons which will be discussed in detail, herbs could be sold legally if they were not labeled for use in the treatment of disease. What this means is that advocacy literature containing the most outrageous claims of therapeutic effectiveness could be sold side-by-side with the drugs, so long as it was not part of the official labeling. To protect the author, most such books and pamphlets carry a carefully worded disclaimer indicating that the reader should refrain from testing any of the suggested remedies but, instead, should consult a physician on all matters pertaining to drugs and therapy. The consumer is thus taunted with information he is warned not to apply!

Voluminous is too conservative a word to apply to the existing quantities of this kind of promotional literature. Staggering is a better term. These modern herbals range from small, cheaply printed, paper-covered pamphlets dealing with single or, at most, small groups of drugs to large, elaborately produced, comprehensive studies in fine bindings with attractive art work and numerous color plates. Some combine herbal lore with astrology. Others, in an obvious attempt to cultivate the interest of drug abusers, emphasize plant substances with mind-altering properties. Still others slant their coverage toward certain groups such as women, vegetarians, youth, the aged, or the outdoorsman. Another type of promotional literature may be viewed as developing from the now discredited "American school of eclectic medicine" in which special attention was given to plant remedies. This has been characterized[1] as "the apotheosis of the old grandmother and witch-doctor systems of treatment."

Practically all these writings recommend large numbers of herbs for the treatment of a variety of ailments based on hearsay, folklore, and tradition; in fact, the only criterion which seems to be rigorously avoided is scientific evidence. Some are so comprehensive and so indiscriminate that they appear to recommend everything for anything. While such lack of judgment should be deplored, it is not nearly so potentially harmful as the many instances where downright dangerous, even deadly poisonous herbs are recommended, usually on the basis of some outdated reference or a misunderstanding of the facts.

Particularly insidious is the myth perpetrated by these promoters that there is something almost *magical* about herbal drugs which prevents them—in their natural state—from inflicting harm on living organisms. Think how completely false this argument is! Even those unfamiliar with the execution of Socrates by poison hemlock more than two thousand years ago are probably not inclined to collect and eat wild mushrooms indiscriminately.

To understand plant drugs completely, we need to know their botany, chemistry, and pharmacology. Few modern herbalists possess such a comprehensive background. Therefore, they rely heavily on outdated writings and without benefit of modern scholarship, transmit the opinions and recommendations of authors who long ago ceased to be authorities. We do not take our automobiles to the livery stable to be serviced; neither should we depend on the 16th century herbalist John Gerard or the 17th century apothecary-astrologer Nicholas Culpeper for modern therapeutic advice. Culpeper's writings are full of astrological explanations for the efficacy of various drugs (which may explain his renewed popularity in the "Age of Aquarius").

However, present-day commentators on Culpeper's writings seem to know even less than he did. One of them[2] tells us that lily-of-the-valley (*Convallaria majalis* L.) ". . . not being poisonous, does not leave any harmful results if it is taken over a long period." Yet all modern authorities characterize the plant as poisonous, and convallatoxin, the principal glycoside contained in it, is regarded as the most toxic cardiac glycoside in existence.[3]

Similar misstatements are not confined to commentaries on Culpeper. Aikman's attractive compilation of folk medicine[4] features photographs of a Virginia woman brewing up an oversized kettle of comfrey leaves to make "a sweet tea for calming coughs and stomach ulcers." This, in spite of evidence that comfrey contains several hepatotoxic pyrrolizidine alkaloids shown to produce cancer of the liver in small animals.[5] Gibbons[6] gives us a recipe for coltsfoot cough drops and says he drinks a medicinal tea made from that plant for "pure pleasure." Coltsfoot also contains a carcinogenic pyrrolizidine alkaloid, senkirkine.[7] Writing in 1977, A. and S. McPherson[8] recommended iced sassafras tea as a "great summer drink" and even give us a recipe for sassafras jelly. Yet, since 1960, sassafras oil and its major constituent, safrole, have been banned as flavoring agents because of their carcinogenicity.[9] A large number of therapeutic uses for pokeroot are described by Leek[10] with no mention of the fact that it is so poisonous that persons drinking a single cup of tea made from it have required hospitalization.[11] Candy lovers eating large amounts of licorice have also become seriously ill,[12] but F. and V. Mitton tell us it has "the greatest value in cough medicine" without a word of warning.[13] The list could go on and on. Enough examples have been cited to demonstrate the lack of critical evaluation in the current herbal literature—and the wisdom of reasoned skepticism.

This brings us to a discussion of another of the tenets of modern herbalism: the dogma that whole drugs—that is, leaves or roots or seeds or the like—have physiological properties different from the active constituents isolated from the same plant parts. This, of course, is a fallacy. While certain plants do contain a large number of active principles and the observed effects following administration will be a combination of all of them, these various principles usually display activities which are qualitatively similar, if not quantitatively identical.

For example, digitalis, the dried leaf of *Digitalis purpurea* L., has long been used in the treatment of congestive heart failure. It contains approximately 30 different glycosides which possess some cardiotonic properties. Two of them, digitoxin and gitalin (really a mixture of several glycosides), are isolated from the leaf and marketed individually as commercially important drugs. All three products, digitalis, digitoxin and gitalin, are used in the same way for treatment of the same disease, namely, congestive heart failure. They differ in potency, in time of onset, and in duration of activity, but they affect the heart in the same way and are therefore qualitatively similar.

Countless other examples could be given. Opium and its principal alkaloid, morphine, produce similar physiological effects. So do cinchona bark and quinine, peppermint leaf and peppermint oil, coffee and caffeine, and wheat germ oil and vitamin E. To be sure, some natural products contain two or more principles with different activities, but these are ordinarily supplementary, not antagonistic. Cod liver oil contains appreciable quantities of both vitamins A and D. These vitamins can be isolated, either from this or other sources, and administered separately at the same dosage with precisely the same effect as that of the natural mixture in the oil. Again, because it is important: remember that *herbs and other drugs exhibit the same types of activity as do the active principles isolated from them.*

Another myth perpetrated by many promoters of herbal therapy is that "natural" products — organic chemicals synthesized in nature by metabolic processes in plants and animals — possess an innate superiority over the same product produced in the chemical laboratory. Such claims at times actually border on mysticism, but then herbs have long been linked by some with astrological phenomena.

Anyone with a knowledge of biology, biochemistry, or even history will recognize that this vitalistic doctrine which draws a sharp distinction between inorganic and organic materials is nothing new. It was completely discredited more than 150 years ago when the German chemist Friedrich Wöhler succeeded in producing the natural organic compound urea from a solution of inorganic ammonium cyanate. When writers show their ignorance of the significance of this event, the wise reader must question the validity of other aspects of their writing as well.

This ignorance still exists today: there is no difference in the vitamin C, for example, obtained from natural biosynthetic processes in rose hips, or by synthetic processes in the laboratory of a chemical manufacturer. The word "natural" applied to such materials identifies only a source and does not imply a degree of superiority or inferiority. However, on the labels of various drugs and vitamins, it does indicate that the consumer may expect to pay several times the normal price for such an item.

Another term much misused in recent writings on herbs is "organic." Applied to a wide variety of "health foods," it denotes that the product was grown under conditions utilizing only natural fertilizers, such as manure, and that no pesticides of any type were applied to it. In some ways this is an extension of the vitalistic doctrine just discussed. Plant physiologists have known for years that plants have no mechanism for differentiating whether nutrients such as calcium, potassium, and nitrogen are derived from organic or inorganic sources, provided they are in a form the plant can assimilate. If anything, the organic forms are less readily available and may have to be acted upon by soil microorganisms before they can be utilized by the plant. Thus, if rapid, profuse growth is desired (as is normally the case) *inorganic or synthetic fertilizers which provide nutrients in a readily available form have a definite advantage.*

Pesticide residues may, of course, pose health hazards if present in sufficient concentrations. Fortunately, most can be removed by proper cleansing, and for those which cannot, appropriate limits of safety have been established. Since exactly the same problem exists with other elements in our environment which we consume every day in huge quantities — including air and water — there would seem to be much less cause for concern about residues on food products. Besides, the typical consumer has absolutely no way of knowing whether the item he has purchased is "organic" or not. All he knows is that he has paid a premium for something which was probably misrepresented.

At this point, you may ask, "If so many of the herbal remedies have little or no value, or may even be dangerous to a person's health, why have they become so very popular in recent years? Why do so many people, especially those who are unusually health-conscious, continue to demand and use them?" The answer lies, at least partly, in the so-called *placebo effect.*

"Placebo" comes from the Latin "I will please" and refers to a drug which provides relief for the patient through mental processes rather than through any physiological effect on his disorder. The placebo effect is thus a physiological improvement brought about by a psychological mechanism. Mind over matter, is a simpler way of putting it. A placebo does for you what you think it will do.

Scientific studies have shown that placebos actually work about one-third of the time.[14] They were found to be effective for the relief of severe postoperative wound pain, cough, drug-induced mood changes, angina pain, headache, seasickness, and the common cold in an average of 35% of these patients. More interesting was the observation that placebos work even better when the goal of therapy is some change in behavior (drowsiness, alertness), in subjective sensation (pain or discomfort), or in a response controlled by the endocrine glands or by the autonomic nervous system (blood pressure, acid stomach, asthmatic breathing). Since many of the conditions for which herbal treatment is commonly used fall into these categories, it is completely understandable why some people find them to be of some value, at least some of the time.

Discussing the placebo effect brings me to why the various

herbal materials in homeopathic medicine are not mentioned in this book. Homeopathy is a system of medicine proposed by Samuel Hahnemann early in the 19th century which hypothesizes that disease is cured by remedies which produce symptoms in a healthy subject resembling the disease in question. However, and this is very important, the cure takes place only when the medicine is administered in such small amounts as to fail to produce the symptoms. Hahnemann based the latter principle on the never-proven assertion that in illness the body is enormously more sensitive to drugs than in health. It led to claims that doses as small as 0.000001 grain (approximately 0.000000065) gram of a medicament could be effective in curing disease. Indeed, such dilutions were referred to as "high potencies."

Practitioners of conventional medicine scoffed at such wild claims, and they still do. One critic versified his objections[15]:

> The homeopathic system, sir, just suits me to a tittle,
> It proves of physic, anyhow, you cannot take too little;
> If it be good in all complaints to take a dose so small,
> It surely must be better still, to take no dose at all.

The interest in unconventional medicine developed during recent years has also extended to homeopathy. Many modern herbals quote homeopathic uses for various drugs. Thoughtful consideration tells us that whatever it may be, the system of homeopathy has no relation whatever to the effective use of drugs of any kind. Probably the best that can be said about this now discredited treatment is that it demonstrates the therapeutic value of the placebo effect.

This book is designed to help consumers decide for themselves, on the basis of the most recent scientific evidence, whether an herb they have considered taking for a particular condition is 1) really potentially useful, 2) essentially without value (except for its possible "placebo effect"), or 3) potentially hazardous, for one reason or another. Hazards, however, should not be thought of simply in terms of toxicity. To some extent, all self-treatment with herbs or any other kind of medication is potentially hazardous because it may cause the patient to neglect conditions which could respond to timely professional therapy but if neglected, could result in serious health problems. Then, too, there is always the hazard to the patient's pocketbook.

For all of the reasons given above, you are less likely to receive good value for money spent in the field of herbal medicine than in almost any other.

REFERENCES

1. M. Fishbein: Fads and Quackery in Healing. Blue Ribbon Books, New York, 1932, p. 31.
2. C. F. Leyel: Culpeper's English Physician & Complete Herbal. Wilshire Book Co., N. Hollywood, Calif., 1972, p. 72.
3. G. Baumgarten: Die Herzwirksamen Glykoside. VEB Georg Thieme, Leipzig, 1963, p. 67.
4. L. Aikman: Nature's Healing Arts. National Geographic Society, Washington, D.C., 1977, pp. 30–31.
5. N. R. Farnsworth: American Journal of Pharmaceutical Education 43: 242, 1979.
6. E. Gibbons: Stalking the Healthful Herbs (Field Guide Ed.). David McKay Co., New York, 1970, pp. 31–32.
7. I. Hirono, H. Mori, and C. C. J. Culvenor: Gann 67: 125–129, 1976.
8. A. McPherson and S. McPherson: Wild Food Plants of Indiana. Indiana University Press, Bloomington, 1977, pp. 99–101.
9. A. B. Segelman, F. P. Segelman, J. Karliner, and R. D. Sofia: Journal of the American Medical Association 236: 477, 1976.
10. S. Leek: Herbs: Medicine & Mysticism. Henry Regnery Co., Chicago, 1975, pp. 198–199.
11. W. H. Lewis and P. R. Smith: Journal of the American Medical Association 242: 2759–2760, 1979.
12. J. W. Conn, D. R. Rovner, and E. L. Cohen: Ibid. Vol. 205, 1968, pp. 492–496.
13. F. and V. Mitton: Mitton's Practical Modern Herbal, W. Foulsham & Co. Ltd., London, 1976, p. 104.
14. M. C. Gerald: American Pharmacy NS19(5): 246, 1979.
15. United States Magazine, and Democratic Review, Vol. 22, p. 418 (1848). In M. Kaufman: Homeopathy in America, The Johns Hopkins Press, Baltimore, 1971, p. 30.

2

LAWS AND REGULATIONS

Herbs abounded in the old-time drugstore. The pharmacist used them mostly to prepare various kinds of solutions and extracts which were then mixed with other ingredients to fill prescriptions. During the past few decades, these drugs in their handsome glass-labeled bottles gradually disappeared from the shelves of the pharmacy, replaced largely by packages of pre-fabricated medicines. Some shops retained a few, along with fancy glass globes of colored water, for show, not for use.

Part of the reason for this change is obvious. Pharmaceutical manufacturers could prepare medicines better, more accurately, and cheaper than any individual could. Not so obvious are the complicated laws and regulations which also exerted great influence on the disappearance of crude drugs from the pharmacy. Not that they disappeared from commerce; far from it. They were simply moved to the so-called health food stores where they continue to exist in great variety and to be sold in enormous quantity. In 1985, the sale of herbs and herb teas in such establishments amounted to more than $190 million, a figure that has remained substantially unchanged for the last several years. Though less than in preceding years, the sale of books explaining the use of herbs and similar products totaled an additional $33 million in 1985. Let's look at the laws and regulations which helped to create this entire situation.

The original Food and Drugs Act of 1906 was, at the time, a bold step forward. It effectively abolished the patent medicine and meat-packing frauds which, thanks to sensational journalism, had been the main causes of the public pressure which led to eventual reform. The Act prohibited adulterated or misbranded drugs but did not deal with the safety or efficacy of the drugs themselves. Those matters were really not addressed for a third of a century.

In the late 1930's, public opinion was again mobilized, this time by the Elixir-of-Sulfanilamide tragedy in which more than 100 persons were fatally poisoned by a newly marketed drug product. As a result, the 1938 Federal Food, Drug, and Cosmetic Act was passed. It required that all drugs sold in this country be proven safe. This Act was subsequently amended in 1962. Since the Drug Amendments of 1962 followed extensive Congressional investigations of the drug industry led by Senator Estes Kefauver, they are still commonly referred to as the Kefauver-Harris Amendments. They required that *all drugs marketed in the United States after 1962 be proven both safe and effective.*

The procedure used since 1938 to make certain of new drug safety was known as a New Drug Application. That title soon became abbreviated to NDA. Something now had to be done so that those drugs already proven safe through the NDA mechanism were also proven effective. Approximately 4000 different drug formulations, representing about 300 different chemical entities, fell into the category of drugs actually being sold, and another 3000 formulations were covered by NDA's but were not actively marketed.

Lacking the resources to tackle this gigantic task itself, the Federal Food and Drug Administration (FDA) turned for help in 1962 to the Division of Medical Sciences of the National Academy of Sciences — National Research Council. They, in turn, organized a "Drug Efficacy Study" which lasted nearly seven years and finally culminated in a report to the FDA in 1969. Our interest here is largely in drugs which may be purchased without a physician's prescription, so-called over-the-counter (OTC) drugs. The study covered 420 of the estimated 350,000 such products and declared that only one-quarter of the 420 examined were effective. These findings pointed out the need for a more comprehensive review of the efficacy of all OTC drugs, applying identical standards to each. Obviously, it would be impossible to study all of the estimated one-third million products, so it was decided to examine only their 200 active ingredients.

A further obstacle needed to be overcome. Some of the older drugs had been "grandfathered" under both the 1938 Act and the 1962 Amendments since they were covered by the original 1906 Food and Drugs Act. How could the FDA remove these drugs from the market? Even if they were proven ineffective, they were apparently immune from the "effective" requirement established at the later dates.

The FDA reached these grandfathered drugs by what can only be described as an extremely innovative application of administrative law.[1] The agency simply declared that a drug would be considered misbranded if the manufacturer made any claims for it which were not in accord with the findings of one of 17 panels set up in 1972 to review the efficacy of the active ingredients of all OTC drugs. In other words, a particular drug, even though exempt from proofs of safety and efficacy under existing laws, was barred from commerce if any unsubstantiated claim was made as part of the labeling that it was "good" for anything, that is, effective for the treatment of a disease state. The word *label* is very broadly interpreted to include not only the words printed on the container or package but also any literature accompanying it, such as a package insert.

In their search for proof of efficacy of the various OTC drugs, the 17 panels, each of which concerned itself with a different class of therapeutic agents, had a number of potential sources of information.[2] Neither testimonials nor market success were considered reliable criteria. This left in vitro tests (tests conducted outside the patient or any living organism) and various kinds of clinical trials (on patients) as the most acceptable methods.

Relatively simple in vitro tests may be suitable for the evaluation of a small number of certain drugs. For example, antacids can be mixed with acid to determine their neutralizing capacity. However, to prove the safety and efficacy of most therapeutic agents, pharmacological studies are necessary. They are ordinarily begun in small animals and continued with increasing complexity all the way through a series of so-called randomized, double-blind clinical trials in human beings. That simply means that some patients selected at random receive the drug while others are given a placebo; neither group knows what they are taking. The results are evaluated by a physician who is also unaware of who is getting what treatment, and after statistical analysis of the data, a judgment is made of the drug's effectiveness.

Such studies, particularly the complex clinical trials, are extremely expensive. Estimates vary, but a 1978 study[3] placed the total cost of developing a single new chemical compound for drug use at more than $50 million! A large part of this figure would certainly be the cost of testing the compound to establish its safety and efficacy as required in the New Drug Application.

Obviously, no company is going to make this kind of investment unless there is a reasonable expectation that it will be able to recover its costs and also show a profit. Since patent protection, now limited to a maximum of 17 years, begins in the very early stages of development of a drug, not when it is approved for marketing by the FDA, about 90% of the new drugs currently introduced have a remaining patent life of less than 11 years. The old "plant" drugs, some of which have been known and used for centuries, do not even qualify for this degree of protection. For this reason, the pharmaceutical industry has shown little interest in sponsoring studies on them, and the safety and efficacy of most herbal remedies remain unproven. Remember, too, that the panels did not necessarily review a drug unless requested to do so by a manufacturer or some other interested party who was then asked to provide quantities of supporting data. To date, many of the older plant drugs have yet to undergo such official scrutiny, while fiscal constraints have caused the independent (non-FDA) panels to be abandoned for further reviews.

This has led to the situation I mentioned before in which practically all herbal remedies have been removed from the shelves of pharmacies and from the supervision of knowledgeable pharmacists. They have now migrated to the "health food" stores where they are sold under the guise of herbs, teas, health foods, food supplements, nutritional products, etc., labeled only with the name of the product. No claim of effectiveness for any condition appears on the label of such containers nor in any leaflet or advertisement which directly accompanies the drug. Any such claim would cause the product to be declared misbranded and render it subject to confiscation. How then does the uninformed consumer learn the uses of the various herbs? Sales people generally avoid recommendations (especially if the customer looks like a law-enforcement official), since such activity could result in a charge of unlicensed practice of medicine. However, the clerks in "health food" stores or the catalogs of mail-order establishments will refer interested persons to a large selection of books, pamphlets, and charts which list the drugs and describe their supposed uses. Some of these information sources are quite broad in scope and are called herbals or natural-medicine books. Others limit their coverage to a single drug or therapeutic class of drugs. Still others list the various diseases or conditions which require treatment and then recommend specific remedies. In this way, current laws and regulations requiring that OTC drugs be proven safe and effective prior to marketing are circumvented.

Labeling a package only with the common name of a drug has some very serious drawbacks aside from the omitted information on utility. The popular names of plants are not only numerous but inexact. Used without a qualifying adjective, the term "snake-root" applies to at least six different plants including *Actaea alba* (l.) Mill., *Aristolochia serpentaria* L., *Asarum canadense* L., *Cimicifuga racemosa* (L.) Nutt., *Eupatorium rugosum* Houtt., and *Senecio aureus* L. Several modifying adjectives are also used to denote these or other species. Thus we have black snakeroot, button snakeroot, Canada snakeroot, corn snakeroot, heart snakeroot, Indian snakeroot, large snakeroot, prairie snakeroot, rattle snakeroot, Sampson's snakeroot, seneca (senega or seneka) snakeroot, Texas snakeroot, Virginia snakeroot, and white snakeroot, among others. When I see any plant material labeled snakeroot, I feel like a rider for the Pony Express watching the last telegraph pole being placed in position on the California line. It's depressing!

We see packages labeled oriental ginseng, wild red American ginseng, Korean ginseng, Tienchi-ginseng, Chinese ginseng, and ginseng ad infinitum and ad nauseam, often with no indication of the botanical origin of the plant material inside. We see mistletoe on an herb tea label and wonder whether it is from the European species (*Viscum album* L.) or the American, since the term could refer to as many as 200 different species of the genus *Phoradendron*. When it comes to gotu kola (which does not contain any cola), and Fo-ti-tieng®, which is not the same as fo-ti, the situation becomes dangerously confusing.

The only answer to this herbal Tower of Babel is to require that the scientific name, that is, the Latin binomial, of the plant appear on the labels of all herbs. As a matter of fact, the American Society of Pharmacognosy has recommended to the FDA that in addition to the scientific name, the label should indicate the part(s) of the plant represented, the country of origin, and a specific lot number which could be related to a voucher specimen maintained for reference purposes. That would solve the identity problem; questions concerning safety, efficacy, and potency would still remain, of course.

One unfortunate part of this whole situation is that at least some of the drugs of natural origin which must legally be sold in this manner without any indication of use are no doubt safe and do possess useful therapeutic properties. We know this from the continued widespread use of these products in countries other than the United States. This is especially true in those countries which are technologically advanced, such as West Germany, but which have more realistic drug laws and regulations, at least in reference to some of the ancient and honorable plant drugs.

One such drug is valerian, the dried rhizome and roots (underground parts) of *Valeriana officinalis* L., which has been valued as a tranquilizing agent for more than one thousand years. It enjoyed official status in the United States for 150 years, and was included in *The United States Pharmacopeia* (U.S.P.) from 1820 to

1942 and in *The National Formulary* from 1942 to 1950. It is still available in pharmacies in the form of a tincture, but the manufacturer has indicated that it would probably drop this product rather than spend the time and money necessary to prove its safety and efficacy — after ten centuries of use.

In contrast to the limited availability of valerian in this country, more than 100 different proprietary drug products containing it or its active principles are currently marketed in Germany. Research carried out there in recent years has established the chemical identity of the constituents responsible for its sedative properties, and these so-called "valepotriates" have been isolated, formulated, and sold as drugs. Valerian and the valepotriates have a significant advantage over synthetic tranquilizers in that their effects are not synergistic with (are not unusually potentiated by) alcohol. It is indeed unfortunate that this useful drug is primarily available in the United States as a foul-smelling tincture or bitter herbal tea instead of a more palatable form. And this is entirely a result of present laws and regulations governing the sale of drugs in this country.

So much for the past and present. What about the future? Fortunately, there are some hopeful signs that this extremely negative legal and regulatory situation in the field of herbal medicine will not continue indefinitely. The ground swell of consumer enthusiasm for all things natural, including herbs, sometimes referred to as the "green wave," may develop enough influence to induce needed changes.[4]

A very encouraging development is currently taking place in Canada. An Expert Advisory Committee on Herbs and Botanical Preparations has issued a report containing several significant recommendations.[5] The most important of these would establish a new class of drugs designated "Folklore Medicines." These would include herbal remedies demonstrated to be safe, but the efficacy of which was not necessarily proven by standard methods applicable to other drugs. This is a very significant deviation from previous policy. Safety testing is a relatively inexpensive process. Proof of effectiveness, on the other hand, may require expenditures approaching $100 million. Since the latter would not be required, many of the old-time herbal remedies could return to the drug market with labeled statements of efficacy supported only by folkloric claims. Other desirable recommendations of the Committee would require that all such products be appropriately labeled and that standards of quality be developed and maintained.

This proposal seems to be a most sensible one, and, if adopted in Canada, should provide a real stimulus to the rational development of the field of herbal medicine. Whether the creation of a special class of herbal drugs, marketed without absolute proof of clinical efficacy, would be feasible in the United States, is a matter open to question. Product liability laws and the litigious climate prevailing in this country would seem to militate against enactment of such a plan, in spite of its many attractive features.

Still, climates are subject to change. If herbal enthusiasts are able to exert sufficient influence, perhaps appropriate legislation could be developed and enacted. Perhaps interested consumers will be able to convince their elected representatives that we should not be satisfied with a we-don't-know answer to the questions of whether catnip really has a useful sedative effect, or if garlic actually reduces high blood pressure, or if ginseng definitely increases resistance to disease. The only way to stimulate the necessary research required to answer such questions definitely is to make it financially profitable to obtain the answers. Easing the unnecessarily rigid standards for marketing plant drugs long in use as folk remedies, is, in my opinion, the best way to accomplish this objective. Personally, I look toward the herbal future with interest, enthusiasm, and modest optimism.

REFERENCES

1. D. R. Harlow: Food, Drug, Cosmetic Law Journal 32: 248–272, 1977.
2. M. C. Gerald: American Pharmacy NS19(5): 18–22, 1979.
3. Anon.: Tile & Till 64: 13, 1978–79.
4. V. E. Tyler: Economic Botany 40: 279–288, 1986.
5. Report of the Expert Advisory Committee on Herbs and Botanical Preparations. Minister of Natural Health and Welfare, Canada, 1986, 17 pp.

3

HERBS AND RELATED REMEDIES

ALFALFA

Anything green that grew out of the mould
Was an excellent herb to our fathers of old.
Rudyard Kipling
"Our Fathers of Old," Stanza 1

Apparently our fathers of more recent vintage were the ones to ascribe therapeutic value to this plant. It is still difficult to understand how alfalfa, or lucerne as it is known in Britain, ever gained a reputation as a medicinal herb. The leaves and flowering tops of *Medicago sativa* L. are not discussed in any of the classic American scientific works on natural drugs.[1,2] Even Grieve's *A Modern Herbal*, a comprehensive work of English origin, scarcely mentions the plant.[3] Of course, this perennial member of the family Leguminosae is one of our most common, cultivated forage plants, being fed to animals either as hay or in a dehydrated form.

Travelers may be familiar with the odor and taste of alfalfa and not even know it. Anyone who has driven Interstate Highway 80 across Nebraska during the summer months and passed through Lexington and Cozad (the alfalfa capital of the world) has noted the peculiar green haze in the air and has smelled the pungent dust from the enormous alfalfa dehydrating plants which abound in that area.

Apparently someone in the recent past decided that if cattle could grow strong and healthy by eating alfalfa, the plant must have therapeutic value for human beings. Consequently, the herb is now widely advocated for consumption in the form of a tea or as tablets or capsules of the dried plant itself for a variety of ailments. We read testimonials to the efficacy of alfalfa tea in the cure of various types of arthritic conditions including rheumatoid arthritis. Advocates also tell us that large quantities of alfalfa tablets taken before meals will prevent the absorption of cholesterol, thus benefiting our arterial blood flow and especially our heart.[4] Claims are made for the effectiveness of the tea in treating diabetes[5] and in stimulating the appetite and acting as a general tonic.

Scientific or clinical evidence in support of these claims is scanty or totally lacking. There is one report that saponins of alfalfa root, which is not the part of the plant generally used, prevented an expected increase in plasma cholesterol in monkeys. But counterbalancing this is evidence that alfalfa saponins are hemolytic and may interfere with the utilization of vitamin E.[6]

Because of its importance as an animal feed, alfalfa has been the subject of numerous and detailed chemical analyses. They have revealed the presence, in addition to the aforementioned saponins, of such constituents as fiber, protein, fats, minerals (calcium, phosphorus, iron, etc.), organic acids, vitamin K_1, a small amount of vitamin C, various pigments including chlorophyll, and the like.[7] While some of these compounds do possess minor physiological activities, none is of significant therapeutic value, at least in the amount present in reasonable quantities of the herb. Considering the absolute lack of any proof of their utility in human medicine, alfalfa tablets which presently may be purchased three or four for a penny are still a bad buy. If you enjoy the taste of alfalfa sprouts in salads, they are refreshing and generally harmless, so feel free to eat them, at least in moderation.

There is good reason to insert the words "in moderation" in the last sentence. Since 1981, it has been recognized that eating very large quantities of alfalfa seeds daily could produce reversible blood abnormalities (pancytopenia) in human beings.[8] More recent studies have shown that systemic lupus erythematosus (SLE), an inflammatory connective tissue disease, can be induced in normal monkeys by feeding alfalfa seeds or sprouts.[9] Also, persons suffering from clinically inactive SLE may have that condition reactivated on taking quantities of alfalfa tablets.[10] It seems likely that a nonprotein amino acid, L-canavanine, contained in alfalfa may play a role in causing the blood abnormalities and in inducing or reactivating SLE in persons having a predisposition to that condition. These latter individuals should be very cautious about consuming any alfalfa product, and since predisposition may not always be recognized, moderation seems generally advisable.

REFERENCES

1. H. W. Felter and J. U. Lloyd: King's American Dispensatory, 18th Ed., Vols. 1–2. The Ohio Valley Company, Cincinnati, 1898 and 1900.

2. H. W. Youngken: Textbook of Pharmacognosy, 6th Ed. The Blakiston Company, Philadelphia, 1943.
3. M. Grieve: A Modern Herbal, vol. 2. Dover Publications, New York, 1971, pp. 501–502.
4. M. Bricklin: The Practical Encyclopedia of Natural Healing. Rodale Press Inc., Emmaus, Pennsylvania, 1976, pp. 28–29, 202–203.
5. R. Adams and F. Murray, Health Foods. Larchmont Books, New York, 1975, pp. 145–147.
6. A. Y. Leung: Encyclopedia of Common Natural Ingredients Used in Food, Drugs, and Cosmetics, John Wiley & Sons, New York, 1980, pp. 15–17.
7. P. H. List and L. Hörhammer, Eds.: Hagers Handbuch der Pharmazeutischen Praxis, 4th Ed., Vol. 5. Springer-Verlag, Berlin, 1976, pp. 732–734.
8. M. R. Malinow, E. J. Bardana, Jr., and S. H. Goodnight, Jr.: Lancet I: 615, 1981.
9. M. R. Malinow, E. J. Bardana, Jr., B. Pirofsky, S. Craig, and P. McLaughlin: Science 216: 415–417, 1982.
10. J. L. Roberts and J. A. Hayashi: New England Journal of Medicine 308: 1361, 1983.

ALOE

. . . the public must learn how to cherish the nobler and rarer plants, and to plant the aloe . . .

Margaret Fuller

lthough she was thinking of the plant in another connection when she wrote the above lines, Margaret Fuller's advice about aloe may be taken quite literally by those seeking a handy, homegrown remedy for minor burns, abrasions, and other skin irritations. There is a vast folk literature indicating that the fresh gel or mucilage of *Aloe barbadensis* Mill. (family Liliaceae), otherwise known as *A. vera* (L.) Webb & Berth. or *A. vulgaris* Lam., promotes wound healing on external application. It has also been taken internally for a variety of maladies.[1,2]

A continuing source of confusion to persons interested in herbs is the fact that aloe is the source of two products that are completely different in their chemical composition and their therapeutic properties but which have very similar names that are sometimes interchanged. Aloe (aloe vera) gel or mucilage is a thin, clear, jellylike material obtained from the so-called parenchymal tissue making up the inner portion of aloe leaves. It is prepared from the leaf by various procedures, all of which involve its separation not only from the inner cellular debris, but, especially, from specialized cells known as pericyclic tubules that occur just beneath the epidermis or rind of these same leaves.[3] Such cells contain a bitter yellow latex or juice that is dried to produce the pharmaceutical product known as aloe, an active cathartic.

Aloe gel (mucilage) is used both externally and internally for its wound-healing properties and as a general tonic or cure-all. This is the aloe product commonly incorporated in a wide variety of nonlaxative drug and cosmetic products. Aloe latex or juice, usually in its dried form, is employed as a potent cathartic. Unfortunately, the mechanical separation processes employed are often not completely effective. So aloe gel is sometimes contaminated with aloe latex, thus inducing an unwanted laxative effect following consumption of the so-called gel. In addition, advertisements prepared by copywriters who do not understand the vast difference between aloe gel and aloe juice often use the word juice to describe the thin mucilaginous gel.

To confuse matters even more thoroughly, there is still another product called aloe that is entirely different from the two just described. That is the aloe of the Bible, the so-called lignaloes or aloe wood, a fragrant wood from an entirely different plant that was once used as an incense.[4] It has nothing to do with the aloe we are discussing except that some persons try to glamorize aloe gel by incorrectly ascribing to it a biblical origin. The names may be the same but the plants referred to are not. Actually, aloe latex has been used as a laxative for about 18 centuries, but neither it nor aloe gel is referred to in the Bible.

Having disposed of these nomenclatural difficulties, let us return to the use of aloe gel (mucilage) as a wound-healing agent and all-around remedy. While many sources agree that the gel possesses some activity in its fresh state, there is considerable doubt whether this activity is retained during storage. Commercial processors claim that the stability problem has been overcome, and a "stabilized" product is incorporated in a wide variety of preparations, including juices, gels, ointments, creams, lotions, and shampoos.[5] However, recent scientific tests failed to verify any beneficial effects of a "stabilized" aloe vera gel on human cells.[6] Fluid from fresh leaf sources was found to promote significantly the attachment and growth of normal human cells grown in artificial culture. It also enhanced the healing of wounded monolayers of such cells. On the other hand, the "stabilized" commercial product not only failed to induce such effects but actually proved toxic to such cultured cells. The investigators who carried out these studies concluded that commercially prepared aloe vera gel fractions "can markedly disrupt the in vitro attachment and growth of human cells."

Aloe gel (often incorrectly designated "juice") is described in the popular literature as a cleanser, anesthetic, antiseptic, antipyretic, antipruritic, nutrient, moisturizer, vasodilator, and is also said to possess anti-inflammatory properties and to promote cell proliferation. Recommendations for internal use range from the treatment of coughs to constipation; externally it is used primarily for burns, for conditioning the skin, and even for headache. A salesman drinks it to "detoxify" his system. One Arkansas physician applied it to relieve the symptoms of poison ivy.[7]

Although the cathartic anthraquinone glycosides that comprise the active principles of aloe latex or juice have been rather thoroughly studied both chemically and pharmacologically, the constituents of aloe gel or mucilage are less well known.[8] None of the sugars, polysaccharides, amino acids, enzymes and other proteins, inorganic salts, traces of vitamins, or large amounts of water that constitute aloe gel can account for the therapeutic properties attributed to it. Still, the impressive body of folklore attesting to its healing properties on external application cannot be denied.[9]

Many people keep a potted aloe plant on the windowsill in the kitchen so that a leaf can be cut off and the freshly exuded gel applied to minor burns. Since the safety of such procedures has never been questioned, it is a therapy which has much to recommend it. Also, the treatment is inexpensive and overcomes the problems of stability and retention of the gel's desirable properties following commercial processing and storage.

REFERENCES

1. J. F. Morton: Economic Botany 15: 311–319, 1961.
2. R. H. Cheney: Quarterly Journal of Crude Drug Research 10: 1523–1530, 1970.
3. D. L. Smothers: Drug & Cosmetic Industry 132(1): 40, 77–80, 1983.
4. J. U. Lloyd: Origin and History of All the Pharmacopeial Vegetable Drugs, Chemicals and Preparations, Vol. 1. The Caxton Press, Cincinnati, 1921, pp. 4–14.
5. J. Flagg: American Perfumer and Aromatics 74(4): 27–28, 61, 1959.
6. W. D. Winters, R. Benavides, and W. J. Clouse: Economic Botany 35: 89–95, 1981.
7. L. Aikman: Nature's Healing Arts, National Geographic Society, Washington, D.C., 1977, p. 10.
8. V. E. Tyler, L. R. Brady, and J. E. Robbers: Pharmacognosy, 8th Ed., Lea & Febiger, Philadelphia, 1981, pp. 60–63.
9. V. E. Tyler: Hoosier Home Remedies, Purdue University Press, West Lafayette, Indiana, 1985, p. 30.

ANGELICA

All parts of the tall, perennial, herbaceous plant *Angelica archangelica* L. (family Umbelliferae) contain a very pleasant-smelling aromatic volatile oil, which probably accounts for the continued use of the root, fruits, and leaves of this and other closely related species of *Angelica* in folk medicine.[1] *Angelica atropurpurea* L. is the one commonly employed in the United States.

The drug has been recommended as an antiflatulant (anti-gas treatment), a diuretic, a diaphoretic (sweat producer), and a counter-irritant. It has also acquired some reputation as an emmenagogue (promotes menstrual flow) and abortifacient. There is no proof that the drug is particularly effective in any of these applications; severe poisoning has resulted from large doses of the root administered in an attempt to induce abortions.

At present, the most important application of angelica root and seed is in the flavoring of various alcoholic beverages. It is a component of a number of herb liqueurs, such as Benedictine and Chartreuse. Together with juniper berries and coriander seed, angelica root is one of the principal flavoring ingredients in gin.[2]

The purplish stems of angelica are sometimes collected and "crystallized" with sugar to make a pleasant-tasting confection. Those who consume them or any other parts of angelica should be aware that the plant contains, in addition to the fragrant volatile oil, a number of furocoumarins, e.g., angelicin, bergapten, imperatorin, and xanthotoxin. On contact with the skin, these so-called psoralens may induce photosensitivity (to the sun), resulting in a kind of dermatitis.[3] Studies have shown that these compounds are photo-carcinogenic (cancer-causing) in laboratory animals and are acutely toxic and mutagenic even in the absence of light. Recently, investigators have concluded that psoralens present risks of such magnitude to man that unnecessary exposure to them (via consumption or contact) should be avoided.[4]

For this reason, the use of angelica as a drug cannot be recommended. To make matters even worse, novice collectors may also confuse angelica with water hemlock (*Cicuta maculata* L.), an extremely poisonous plant.[5]

REFERENCES

1. H. W. Youngken: Textbook of Pharmacognosy, 6th Ed. The Blakiston Co., Philadelphia, 1948, pp. 623–625.

2. E. Guenther: The Essential Oils, Vol. 4. D. Van Nostrand Co., New York, 1950, pp. 553–563.
3. P. H. List and L. Hörhammer, Eds.: Hagers Handbuch der Pharmazeutischen Praxis, 4th Ed., Vol. 3. Springer-Verlag, Berlin, 1972, pp. 88–98.
4. G. W. Ivie, D. L. Holt, and M. C. Ivey: Science 213: 909–910, 1981.
5. W. C. Muenscher: Poisonous Plants of the United States. The Macmillan Co., New York, 1951, p. 175.

APRICOT PITS (LAETRILE)

Fraudulent and ineffective cancer cures are as old as the disease itself, and the intervention of well-meaning but medically naive "politicians" to treat it stems from an early date as well. In 1748, the House of Burgesses of the Commonwealth of Virginia undertook a study of one Mary Johnson's herbal "receipt of curing cancer." As a result of the anecdotal testimony provided, the House voted Mrs. Johnson a reward of 100 pounds. Similarly, in 1964, 56 United States Congressmen cosponsored a resolution, which fortunately failed to pass, authorizing the expenditure of $250,000 for the study of another unproven cancer remedy, krebiozen.[1]

During the 1970's, another fake cancer cure, laetrile, began to be widely promoted and used. In spite of the fact that there existed absolutely no scientific evidence for its therapeutic efficacy, demand for the product became so great that by 1981 the legislatures of some 23 states had legalized its use.[2] This whole sordid history, highlighted by (but not restricted to) Mary Johnson's "receipt," krebiozen, and laetrile, apparently indicates that in the absence of a cure for a terminal disease, desperate people want hope, not facts.

Laetrile®, as originally patented in the United States in 1961, is not the same compound as the one called laetrile today.[3] The former was technically known as mandelonitrile glucuronide, but it was relatively difficult to procure. Consequently, a closely related compound, amygdalin (mandelonitrile β-d-gentiobioside), became the laetrile of commerce. It is also sometimes referred to as vitamin B_{17}, although it is definitely not a vitamin. Amygdalin occurs naturally in a number of plant materials; however, the usual commercial source is the kernel of various varieties of Prunus armeniaca L. (family Rosaceae), commonly referred to as apricot pits. These vary appreciably in their amygdalin or laetrile content which may reach 8%, but the kernels of some wild varieties contain 20 times as much as those of cultivated varieties of apricots. Serious cases of poisoning, especially among children have been reported as a result of eating quantities of these seeds.[4]

Advocates of laetrile therapy for cancer believe that an enzyme, β-glucosidase, capable of breaking down the laetrile to release toxic cyanide, exists in large amounts in tumorous tissue but only in small quantities in the rest of the body. They further hypothesize that another enzyme, rhodanese [sic], which has the ability to detoxify cyanide, is present in normal tissues but deficient in cancer cells. These two factors supposedly combine to effect a selective poisoning of cancer cells by the cyanide released from the laetrile, while normal cells and tissues remain undamaged.[5] Needless to say, no scientific proof of this so-called mechanism of action has ever been presented.

Lacking any proof of safety and efficacy, the Food and Drug Administration banned laetrile from interstate commerce in 1971. However, several state legislatures reacting to political pressures legalized intrastate sale and use of the product. Similar pressures forced the National Cancer Institute in 1980 to begin a clinical study of laetrile in terminal cancer patients.[6] Conducted in collaboration with four major U.S. medical centers, the clinical tests showed that laetrile failed on four counts: it did not make cancer regress; it did not extend the lifespan of cancer patients; it did not improve cancer patients' symptoms; and it did not help cancer patients to gain weight or otherwise become more physically active.[7] Laetrile and natural products containing it, such as apricot pits, were thus found to be "ineffective as a treatment for cancer."

There is no reason to utilize apricot pits for any medical purpose. In fact, there are two good reasons—lack of proven safety and efficacy—for not doing so. Still, as this is written, stories in the popular press would seem to indicate that some gullible people, desiring to cure the incurable, will continue to advocate and to utilize this perniciously fraudulent drug, at least until the next bigger, better, and newer quack cure comes along.

REFERENCES

1. R. N. Grant and I. Bartlett: In Unproven Methods of Cancer Management, American Cancer Society, New York, 1971, pp. 1–2.
2. The Indianapolis Star, Feb. 13, 1981, p. 23.
3. C. Fenselau, S. Pallante, R. P. Batzinger, W. R. Benson, R. P. Barron, E. B. Sheinin, and M. Maienthal: Science 198: 625–627, 1977.
4. J. W. Sayre and S. Kaymakcalan: New England Journal of Medicine 270: 1113–1115, 1964.
5. D. L. Poulson: Herbalist 4(4): 2–5, 1979.
6. T. H. Jukes: Journal of the American Medical Association 242: 719–720, 1979.
7. Science News 119: 293–294, 1981.

ARNICA

The medicinal virtues of arnica were independently discovered by Europeans before the end of the 16th century and by American Indians at an early but uncertain date. Originally, the entire plant including the roots was employed, often internally, for a variety of conditions. Subsequently, the flower heads alone began to be used, either as a tincture (dilute alcoholic solution) or an ointment. The European drug is obtained from *Arnica montana* L.; the American product comes from *Arnica fulgens* Pursh, *A. sororia* Greene, and *A. cordifolia* Hook. All are closely related perennial herbs of the family Compositae with orange-yellow daisylike flower heads. They are native to the meadows and mountainous regions of Europe and America.[1]

Recent writers on herbs recommend the application of arnica externally to reduce the inflammation and pain of bruises, aches and sprains.[2] They often provide directions for the formulation of various arnica preparations intended for such external use.[3] Most discourage internal use of the drug, pointing out its involvement in severe, even fatal, cases of poisoning.

Scientific studies of the effects of alcoholic extracts of arnica on the heart and circulatory system of small animals have verified the folly of using the drug internally for self-medication.[4] Not only did it exhibit a toxic action on the heart, but in addition, it caused very large increases in blood pressure. More recent studies have confirmed arnica's cardiac toxicity.[5]

External application of the drug is quite a different matter. Although widely used as a home remedy for aches and bruises, no one could explain how or why arnica worked, if indeed it did. Sollmann, a respected pharmacologist, even speculated that the main active ingredient in arnica tincture was perhaps the alcohol.[6] Chemical studies isolated and identified large numbers of constituents,[7] but none of them accounted for the drug's reputed anti-inflammatory and analgesic effects.

Finally, in 1981, a report from Germany, where more than 100 different drug preparations containing arnica extract are currently marketed, revealed that certain sesquiterpenoid lactones were the active principles.[5] Helenalin, dihydrohelenalin, as well as esters of these two compounds possess pharmacologic properties which explain a number of the actions of arnica. Besides producing anti-inflammatory and analgesic effects, the compounds are also supposed to display some antibiotic activity. One drawback must be noted however. Helenalin is a kind of allergen and causes contact dermatitis in some persons. If this occurs, the application of arnica should immediately be discontinued.

Although more scientific studies are needed to define more precisely the physiologic properties of helenalin and related compounds in arnica, there seems to be some rationale for its external application to reduce the inflammation and pain of various aches and bruises. This is vividly described in a turn-of-the-century poem about the damage inflicted on a candidate during an overly enthusiastic lodge initiation ceremony:

> The house is full of arnica,
>   And mystery profound;
> We do not dare to run about
>   Or make the slightest sound
>
> We leave the big piano shut
>   And do not strike a note;
> The doctor's been here seven times
>   Since father rode the goat.
>
> He joined the Lodge a week ago—
>   Got in at four A.M.,
> And sixteen brethren brought him home,
>   Though he says he brought them.
> His wrist was sprained and one big rip
>   Had rent his Sunday coat—
> There must have been a lively time
>   When father rode the goat.

REFERENCES

1. A. Osol and G. E. Farrar, Jr.: The Dispensatory of the United States of America, 24th Ed. J. B. Lippincott, Philadelphia, 1947, pp. 98–100.
2. M. Grieve: A Modern Herbal, Vol. 1. Dover Publications, New York, 1971. p. 55.
3. W. H. Hylton, Ed.: The Rodale Herb Book. Rodale Press Book Div., Emmaus, Pa., 1974, pp. 351–352.
4. A. W. Forst: Naunyn-Schmiedebergs Archiv für experimentelle Pathologie und Pharmakologie 201: 242–260, 1943.
5. W. Werner: Deutsche Apotheker Zeitung 121: 199, 1981.
6. T. Sollmann: A Manual of Pharmacology, 7th Ed. W. B. Saunders, Philadelphia, 1948, p. 146.
7. A. Y. Leung: Encyclopedia of Common Natural Ingredients Used in Food, Drugs, and Cosmetics. John Wiley & Sons, New York, 1980, pp. 34–35.

BARBERRY

One of the confusing curiosities of crude drug nomenclature is the fact that barberry or berberis is obtained from plants of the genus *Mahonia* and not from species of *Berberis*. The reason for this is that the several species which yield the rhizome and roots (underground parts) which constitute this drug were once classified as *Berberis* species but are now placed in the genus *Mahonia*. They include *M. aquifolium* (Pursh) Nutt. and *M. nervosa* (Pursh) Nutt., both commonly referred to as Oregon grape. These attractive members of the family Berberidaceae are evergreen shrubs with hollylike leaves and bluish-black berries; *M. aquifolium* is generally taller (3 feet plus) than *M. nervosa* (up to 2 feet). Common barberry, *Berberis vulgaris* L., was not a recognized source of the drug when it had official status, but the bark of its root and stem contains similar active principles and is also used similarly.[1]

Barberry was reportedly used by the American Indians in cases of general debility and to improve the appetite. When the early settlers observed this, they employed the root as a bitter tonic. In addition, it was said to be of value as a treatment for ulcers, heartburn, and stomach problems when given in small doses; large doses have a cathartic effect.[2]

A number of isoquinoline alkaloids, especially berberine, berbamine, and oxyacanthine, account for the physiological activity of barberry. Several of the alkaloids exhibit antibacterial properties, and berberine is also effective against both amoeba and trypanosomes. This alkaloid has some anticonvulsant, sedative, and uterine-stimulant properties as well. Berbamine produces a hypotensive effect (lowers blood pressure).[3]

In spite of these various properties, barberry and its contained alkaloids, of which berberine is the principal one, are not very useful drugs. Including the crude plant material in bitter tonics has been essentially discontinued. Berberine salts continued for some time to be used in eye drops because of their astringent properties, but this, too, has now ceased. There appears to be no reason to recommend barberry for its therapeutic properties. Any serious discussion of the drug belongs more properly in the history books, not in medical books.

REFERENCES

1. A. Osol and G. E. Farrar, Jr., Eds.: The Dispensatory of the United States of America, 24th Ed. J. B. Lippincott, Philadelphia, 1947, pp. 1361–1363.
2. W. H. Hylton, Ed.: The Rodale Herb Book. Rodale Press Book Div., Emmaus, Pa. 1974, pp. 352–353.
3. A. Y. Leung: Encyclopedia of Common Natural Ingredients Used in Food, Drugs, and Cosmetics. John Wiley, New York, 1980, pp. 52–53.

BAYBERRY

The bayberry or wax myrtle plant, *Myrica cerifera* L. of the family Myricaceae, is a large evergreen shrub or small tree widely distributed throughout the eastern and southern United States. It is best known for its small bluish-white berries, the wax from which is used to make the fragrant-smelling bayberry candles popular at Christmas.

In folk medicine, the root bark is administered internally, usually in the form of a warm infusion or tea, for its tonic, stimulant, and astringent properties. It is reputed to be especially valuable in the treatment of diarrhea. In large doses, bayberry bark acts as an emetic due to its irritating action on the stomach. The drug has also been used to increase the secretion of nasal mucus during head colds.[1] Applied in the form of poultices, the root bark is said to be useful in the treatment of chronic, so-called indolent, ulcers. One modern herbalist[2] describes the drug as, "If not absolutely the most useful article in botanic practice, it is certainly nearly so."

The nature of many recent herbal writings may be deduced from books published as recently as 1980[3] which continue to list only those constituents of bayberry originally determined in 1863[1] by analytical procedures now thought extremely primitive. These compounds include an acrid and an astringent resin, tannic acid, gallic acid, and a principle called myricinic acid which has never been characterized chemically.

Recent chemical investigations have identified several interesting chemical compounds in bayberry root bark. Three triterpenes, myricadiol, taraxerol, and taraxerone, are present in the drug plus a flavonoid glycoside myricitrin. Of these compounds, myricadiol has been reported to have mineralocorticoid activity, i.e., it influences sodium and potassium metabolism in the same way as the steroid principles of the adrenal cortex. Myricitrin has been shown to function as a choleretic (stimulates flow of bile) and as an agent toxic to bacteria, paramecia, and sperm.[4]

However, even if bayberry were a useful drug for any particular condition—a hypothesis which remains unproven—its safety, at least in large doses, is still in doubt because of the potential carcinogenic nature of its contained tannin. Injection of bark extracts into rats produced a significant number of malignant tumors during a relatively long-term (78 weeks) experiment.[5] These results raise a question about the safety of bayberry for consumption by human beings. Since the root bark has no proven medicinal value anyway, it seems best to restrict the use of the plant to its berries, whose wax does make nice-smelling candles.

REFERENCES

1. G. M. Hambright: American Journal of Pharmacy 35: 193–202, 1863.
2. R. C. Wren and R. W. Wren: Potter's New Cyclopaedia of Botanical Drugs and Preparations (new ed.) Health Science Press, Hengiscote, England, 1975, p. 30.
3. D. G. Spoerke, Jr.: Herbal Medications. Woodbridge Press Publishing Co., Santa Barbara, Calif., 1980, pp. 29–30.
4. B. D. Paul, G. Subba Rao, and G. J. Kapadia: Journal of Pharmaceutical Sciences 63: 958–959, 1974.
5. G. J. Kapadia, B. D. Paul, E. B. Chung, B. Ghosh, and S. N. Pradhan: Journal of the National Cancer Institute 57: 207–209, 1976.

BETONY

B etony or Wood Betony is one of those medicinal plants once thought to be good for practically everything whose use in folk medicine decreased over the years until it is now thought to be of relatively little value. Its earlier importance is indicated by two old proverbs or sayings: Both the Italian, "Sell your coat and buy betony," and the Spanish, "He has as many virtues as betony," emphasize its former versatility as a remedy.

The drug consists of the dried herb, i.e., the entire overground portion of the plant *Stachys officinalis* (L.) Trevisan, a square-stemmed perennial of the family Labiatae with a rosette of hairy leaves and a spike of pink or purplish flowers which attains a height of up to 3 feet. It is native to the cleared areas and meadows of Europe and is widely cultivated in herb gardens.[1]

In Roman times, the plant was thought to be a sure cure for 47 different diseases. (There is no need to list them because any one you can think of was probably included.) During the Middle Ages, many magical properties, including power against evil spirits, were attributed to betony.[2] Today the drug is still highly valued in folk medicine but principally for its properties as an astringent in treating diarrhea and irritations of the throat, mouth, and gums. An infusion or tea prepared from the leaves is either drunk or used as a gargle or mouthwash, according to the condition being treated.[3]

Betony contains about 15% tannin, which explains its use and its effectiveness as an astringent drug.[4] A Russian study found a mixture of glycosides in the plant, at least one of which was a flavonoid pigment. These glycosides were reported to have hypotensive (lower blood pressure) effects.[5] Although the report requires verification, it might partially explain the supposed effectiveness of betony in treating mild anxiety states and headache.

Still, the only known utility of the drug is its astringent action, due to the tannins, which makes it effective in treating diarrhea and various irritations of the mucous membranes. In normal usage, betony should not cause any notable side effects, but overdosing may result in excessive irritation of the stomach.

REFERENCES

1. M. Stuart, Ed.: The Encyclopedia of Herbs and Herbalism. Grosset and Dunlap, New York, 1979, pp. 266–267.

2. M. Grieve: A Modern Herbal, Vol. 1. Dover Publications, New York, 1971, pp. 97–99.
3. M. Pahlow: Das grosse Buch der Heilpflanzen. Gräfe and Unzer GmbH, Munich, 1979, p. 83.
4. P. H. List and L. Hörhammer, Eds.: Hagers Handbuch der Pharmazeutischen Praxis, 4th Ed., Vol. 6B. Springer-Verlag, Berlin, 1979, pp. 506–507.
5. T. V. Zinchenko and I. M. Fefer: Farmatsevtichnii Zhurnal (Kiev) 17(3): 35–38, 1962.

BLACK COHOSH

Black cohosh consists of the underground parts (rhizome and roots) of the showy North American forest plant *Cimicifuga racemosa* (L.) Nutt. Other scientific names applied to it are *Actaea racemosa* L. and *Macrotys actaeoides* Raf. Its common names are also numerous and include black snakeroot, rattleweed, rattleroot, bugbane, bugwort, and squaw root (not to be confused with blue cohosh).

The drug was introduced into medicine by the American Indians who valued it highly. They boiled the root in water and drank the resulting beverage for a variety of conditions ranging from rheumatism, diseases of women, and debility, to sore throat.[1] It was subsequently used, especially by eclectic physicians, for all these conditions but particularly for so-called uterine difficulties to stimulate the menstrual flow. Black cohosh was one of the principal ingredients in Lydia Pinkham's Vegetable Compound. Modern herbalists recommend it for all of the above ailments and also as an astringent, diuretic, alterative, antidiarrheal, cough suppressant, diaphoretic, etc.[2]

Modern scientific studies designed to identify specific physiological activities in the drug have not been numerous, and most have been carried out abroad. The long-suspected estrogenic effects, based on its use to stimulate menstruation, could not be verified in comprehensive experiments in mice.[3] A steroidal triterpene derivative called actein[4,5] was found to lower blood pressure in rabbits and cats but not in dogs. It produced no hypotensive effects in either normal or hypertensive human beings, although some peripheral vasodilation was observed.

Consequently, none of the purported activities of black cohosh in human beings has been scientifically verified nor has its safety been established. The drug is no longer recognized by *The Unites States Pharmacopeia — The National Formulary* (U.S.P. — N.F.), and its use in medical practice has been discontinued. There appears to be no reason to utilize it — or any preparation containing it — for therapeutic purposes.

REFERENCES

1. J. U. Lloyd: Origin and History of all the Pharmacopeial Vegetable Drugs, Chemicals and Preparations, Vol. 1. The Caxton Press, Cincinnati, 1921, pp. 54–62.

2. R. C. Wren and R. W. Wren: Potter's New Cyclopaedia of Botanical Drugs and Preparations, New Ed. Health Science Press, Hengiscote, England, 1975, p. 89.
3. M. Siess and G. Seybold: Arzneimittel-Forschung 10: 514–520, 1960.
4. E. Genazzani and L. Sorrentino: Nature 194: 544–545, 1962.
5. S. Corsano, G. Piancatelli, and L. Panizzi: Gazzetta Chimica Italiana 99: 915–932, 1969.

BLUE COHOSH

One of the oldest indigenous American plant drugs is blue cohosh, otherwise known as papoose root or squaw root. It consists of the underground parts (roots and rhizomes) of *Caulophyllum thalictroides* (L.) Michx., a perennial herb, purple when young, which has a smooth stem, 1 to 3 feet in height, terminated by a panicle of yellowish green flowers. The mature plant is a peculiar bluish green color and bears dark blue fruits; hence, the name, blue cohosh. It is a member of the family Berberidaceae.[1]

Blue cohosh was introduced into medicine in 1813 by Peter Smith, an "Indian herb doctor." It was said to be employed by the Indians for rheumatism, dropsy, colic, sore throat, cramp, hiccough, epilepsy, hysterics, inflammation of the uterus, etc. Subsequently, it gained a reputation as an antispasmodic, emmenagogue (menstrual flow stimulant), and parturifacient (inducer of labor), as well as a diuretic, diaphoretic, and expectorant. Modern herbals still recommend it for various female conditions, especially as a uterine stimulant, inducer of menstruation, and antispasmodic.[2]

The plant contains a number of alkaloids and glycosides, of which the alkaloid methylcytisine and the glycoside caulosaponin seem to contribute most of the physiological activity. Animal experiments have shown that the actions of methylcytisine resemble those of nicotine.[3] The compound elevates blood pressure and stimulates both respiration and intestinal motility. It is only about 1/40 as toxic as nicotine. Blue cohosh's oxytocic (hastening childbirth) effects are apparently produced by the glycoside caulosaponin, a derivative of the triterpenoid saponin hederagenin.[4,5] Caulosaponin constricts the coronary blood vessels, thus exerting a toxic effect on cardiac muscle, and causes intestinal spasms in small animals.

In view of the presence of such relatively potent principles in the drug, blue cohosh cannot be dismissed as either inactive or harmless. The case for or against using it as self-medication, particularly to stimulate uterine contractions or to induce menstruation, probably rests on the advisability of using any self-selected drug for such purposes. The safety of such treatment is by no means certain. Kingsbury[6] points out that the toxicity of English ivy is probably the result of the presence of a saponin glycoside derived, like caulosaponin, from hederagenin. Discretion dictates that blue cohosh not be used for medical self-treatment.

REFERENCES

1. H. W. Felter and J. U. Lloyd: King's American Dispensatory, 18th Ed., Vol. 1. The Ohio Valley Co., Cincinnati, 1898, pp. 468–472.
2. N. Coon: Using Plants for Healing, 2nd Ed. Rodale Press, Emmaus, Pa., 1979, p. 81.
3. C. C. Scott and K. K. Chen: Journal of Pharmacology and Experimental Therapeutics 79: 334–339, 1943.
4. H. C. Ferguson and L. D. Edwards: Journal of the American Pharmaceutical Association (Scientific Edition) 43: 16–21, 1954.
5. J. McShefferty and J. B. Stenlake: Journal of the Chemical Society 2314–2316, 1956.
6. J. M. Kingsbury: Poisonous Plants of the United States and Canada. Prentice-Hall, Englewood Cliffs, N.J., 1964, pp. 371–372.

BONESET

Names of plants often reveal much information about them. They can also be misleading. There is little difficulty with the scientific name of boneset, *Eupatorium perfoliatum* L. The genus name of this member of the daisy family (Compositae) derives from Mithridates Eupator, ancient king of Pontus, who first used a closely related plant for medicinal purposes. The species designation, *perfoliatum*, refers to the manner in which the erect hairy stem of the hardy perennial herb, which attains a height of about 5 feet and is crowned with heads of white tubular florets, appears to perforate the center of the pairs of oppositely joined leaves. Boneset, the common name, is more likely to lead one astray since the plant was classically employed in the treatment of fevers, not to mend broken bones. But when it is recognized that the old name for dengue was breakbone fever, the derivation becomes clear.[1]

American Indians introduced the use of boneset leaves and flowering tops to the early settlers for the treatment of colds, catarrh, influenza, rheumatism, and all kinds of fevers, including breakbone (dengue), intermittent (malaria), and lake (typhoid). To break up colds and flu, the drug is taken in the form of a hot tea to induce sweating and relieve the associated aches and pains. For loss of appetite, indigestion, and as a general bitter tonic, cold boneset infusion is recommended 30 minutes before meals.[2] In either case, the remedy is a bitter, astringent one with a nauseous taste. The hot version is much more likely to cause vomiting than the cold.[3]

Chemical studies have recently identified some of the constituents of boneset, which include various flavonoid pigments, sterols, and triterpenes.[4-6] Compounds with pronounced therapeutic virtues are apparently absent.

Whatever activity the plant may possess seems to be associated with its nauseant properties which do cause increased perspiration. In view of this singular lack of effectiveness, it seems incredible that the plant held official drug status in this country from 1820 to 1950, even though it was rarely prescribed by physicians, at least during the latter part of that period.[7] Nevertheless, there is presently a revival of interest in the use of boneset among adherents to herbal medicine who employ it primarily to relieve fevers. Although safer and more effective treatments, such as common aspirin, certainly exist, it is comforting to know that the medical literature is essentially devoid of reports of adverse incidents attributed to boneset.[8]

REFERENCES

1. W. H. Hylton, Ed.: The Rodale Herb Book. Rodale Press Book Div., Emmaus, Pa., 1974, pp. 369–371.
2. E. Gibbons: Stalking the Healthful Herbs, Field Guide Ed. David McKay Co., New York, 1970, pp. 27–29.
3. L. Aikman: Nature's Healing Arts: From Folk Medicine to Modern Drugs, National Geographic Soc., Washington, D.C., 1977, pp. 40, 42.
4. H. Wagner, M. A. Iyengar, L. Hörhammer, and W. Herz: Phytochemistry 11: 1504–1505, 1972.
5. W. Herz, S. Gibaja, S. V. Bhat, and A. Srinivasan: Phytochemistry 11: 2859–2863, 1972.
6. X. A. Domínguez, J. A. González Quintanilla, and M. Paulino Rojas: Phytochemistry 13: 673–674, 1974.
7. A. Osol and G. E. Farrar, Jr., Eds.: The Dispensatory of the United States of America, 24th Ed. J. B. Lippincott, Philadelphia, 1947, pp. 461–462.
8. D. M. Baker: Lawrence Review of Natural Products 4: 21–23, 1983.

BORAGE

Eating the leaves and flowers of borage, a hairy annual herb attaining a height of about 2 feet, has long been believed to confer both happiness and courage on the consumer. Indeed, Gerard[1] tells us that such attributes of *Borago officinalis* L. were recorded as early as the first century A.D. when Pliny and Dioscorides observed that these plant parts added to wine made persons glad and merry. In the second century A.D., Galen noted that the leaves possessed diuretic properties and also, when mixed with honey, were useful in treating throat irritations. These recommendations are still being repeated, nearly 2000 years later, by modern herbalists.[2,3]

After such a lengthy period of use, one thing is certain. One need not be concerned about the relative safety of consuming borage. The fresh plant has a somewhat salty taste and its odor is reminiscent of cucumbers. So, if it brings pleasure to the palate and the nose, it may be eaten either raw or cooked, like spinach. Alternatively, one may follow Gibbons' recipes and use it in the form of borage syrup, borage candy, borage jam, or borage jelly.[4] Even borage tea appeals to some.

But if you are expecting truly beneficial medicinal effects from this plant, try something else. Tests carried out in small animals found borage to be practically inert, except for a slight constipating effect attributable to its tannin content.[5] Tannin also accounts for the plant's astringent properties, whereas the presence of mucilage explains its mild expectorant action. The diuretic effects, if any, have been variously attributed to malic acid and to potassium nitrate.[6] Borage does contain appreciable concentrations of mineral salts.

As for the plant's ability to do away with sadness, dullness, and melancholy, we have to remember that the flowers and leaves were first soaked in wine which was then drunk to accomplish this purpose. Sufficient quantities of wine, without the borage, will achieve the same result—temporarily. And borage no more stimulates real courage than the potion in the square green bottle which the Wizard fed to the Cowardly Lion in *The Wizard of Oz*. But the belief has left us with an interesting old Latin verse:

"Ego Borago gaudia semper ago."

Gerard renders this in the English of 1597 as:

"I Borage bring alwaies courage."

In 1950, Hannig[5] summarized our knowledge of the therapeutic utility of borage (in translation):

> In conclusion, the drug certainly will not enrich our materia medica. It may be numbered among the numerous tannin and mucilage containing drugs whose actions are nonspecific.

This statement summarizing the relatively ineffective but nevertheless harmless nature of borage was considered valid by most authorities until quite recently. Then, in 1984, scientists reported the discovery of small amounts of two unsaturated pyrrolizidine alkaloids, lycopsamine and supinidine viridiflorate, in the leaves, stems, and roots of the plant.[7] These compounds are suspected poisons, but the low levels at which they occur in borage may account for the lack of any acute toxicity reports associated with the use of this herb. Until further clarification is obtained, it seems prudent to avoid any excessive or long-term consumption of borage.

REFERENCES

1. J. Gerard: The Herball or Generall History of Plants. John Norton, London, 1597, pp. 652–654.
2. R. C. Wren and R. W. Wren: Potter's New Cyclopaedia of Botanical Drugs and Preparations, New Ed. Health Science Press, Hengiscote, England, 1975, pp. 45–46.
3. W. H. Hylton, Ed.: The Rodale Herb Book. Rodale Press Book Div., Emmaus, Pa., 1976, pp. 371–375.
4. E. Gibbons: Stalking the Healthful Herbs, Field Guide Ed. David McKay Co., New York, 1970, pp. 53–57.
5. E. Hannig: Die Pharmazie 5: 35–40, 1950.
6. H. W. Felter and J. U. Lloyd: King's American Dispensatory, 18th Ed., Vol. 1. The Ohio Valley Co., Cincinnati, 1898, p. 643.
7. K. M. Larson, M. R. Roby, and F. R. Stermitz: Journal of Natural Products 47: 747–748, 1984.

BRAN

Dietary fiber may be defined as all foods eaten by a monogastric (one stomach) animal that reach the large intestine essentially unchanged. This includes cellulose, the skeletal material of plant cell walls, and lignin, the rigid component of peach pits and nut shells, for instance. Together these materials are known as "crude fiber." Add to crude fiber such basically indigestible plant cell contents as gums, mucilages, pectic substances, hemicelluloses, and certain complex polysaccharides, and the total is collectively referred to as "dietary fiber."[1]

A cheap and abundant source of dietary fiber is bran, the coarse outer coat or hull of the grain of wheat, *Triticum aestivum* L. (family Gramineae), separated from the meal or flour by sifting or bolting. Bran may also be obtained from other cereal grains, but then the source must be specified. Bran contains about 26.7% dietary fiber: by comparison, baked beans have 7.27%, boiled carrots 3.7%, and whole peaches 2.28%.[2] Lettuce, which many persons consider as real "roughage," contains only about 0.85% dietary fiber.[3]

Studies carried out in the early 1970's on rural black populations in South Africa showed that persons eating more than 50 grams of dietary fiber per day seemed to be relatively free from appendicitis, diseases of the colon (diverticulosis, polyps, or cancer), and to suffer less from ischemic heart disease (coronary artery disease), diabetes, and hiatus hernia than those persons eating more refined diets containing much smaller amounts of fiber. Interestingly, when the rural blacks moved to the cities and adopted Western habits, including diet, they began to suffer from the same Western diseases.

The beneficial effects of high dietary fiber foods such as bran on various gastrointestinal diseases, including cancer, are thought to come from 1) its ability to dilute, in the large amount of water held by the fiber, any carcinogens which might be present and 2) to decrease the contact time with potentially damaging substances, since the larger stool is expelled more rapidly. Passing stools more easily causes less straining and therefore reduces the frequency of hiatus hernia and hemorrhoids. Although the preventive effects of high-fiber diets in cardiovascular disease and diabetes are somewhat more speculative, these may result from the ability of specific polysaccharides to exert hypocholesteremic (lower cholesterol) and hypoglycemic (lower blood sugar) effects in man.[1]

Another way of expressing these actions is to say that the fiber passes through the gut somewhat like a large wet sponge, absorbing and holding not only water and toxicants but such compounds as bile acids, which in turn might modify cholesterol metabolism. The sponge, due to its great bulk, also increases the size of the stool and decreases the emptying time of the colon.[4]

Bran is commercially available in a variety of forms ranging from the crude material sold in bulk to compressed tablets. Probably the most popular sources in the United States are breakfast cereals; the whole bran types contain about 9 grams of dietary fiber per ounce (28.4 grams) which is approximately one-half cup. Of course, you should remember that bran is only one kind of dietary fiber and that many other varieties are present in such foods as legumes and fruits. Eating these is also desirable.

Although the advantages of a diet high in fiber are based on evidence from epidemiologic, experimental, and clinical studies,[5] it will be many years before all the hypotheses to account for these observations can be thoroughly tested. In the meantime, it is not surprising that opinions are wide-ranging on the amount of dietary fiber to be eaten daily by an adult. At present, the average American diet provides only 2 to 5 grams per day. Recommendations range from 10 grams[6] to as much as 60 grams.[1] An intermediate figure is probably more realistic, but this must be based largely on the individual's tolerance to increased bulk in the diet.

For best results, an increased intake in dietary fiber should be accompanied by a reduction in foods high in sugar, salt, and fat. Where possible, get the dietary fiber from whole-grain cereals and bread, potatoes, vegetables, and fruits. Supplement as necessary with bran. This may not result in "instant health," but there is a good possibility that it may reduce the frequency of certain chronic illnesses.

REFERENCES

1. A. I. Mendeloff: New England Journal of Medicine 297: 811–814, 1977.
2. V. E. Tyler, L. R. Brady, and J. E. Robbers: Pharmacognosy, 8th Ed. Lea & Febiger, Philadelphia, 1981, p. 474.

3. R. G. Marks: Drug Topics 124(15): 20, 1980.
4. P. Gunby: Journal of the American Medical Association 238: 1715–1716, 1977.
5. R. Adams and F. Murray: Health Foods. Larchmont Books, New York, 1975, pp. 33–39.
6. M. A. Krupp and M. J. Chatton: Current Medical Diagnosis and Treatment 1980. Lange Medical Publications, Los Altos, Calif., 1980, pp. 786–787.

BROOM

The tops of *Cytisus scoparius* (L.) Link, a large, yellow-flowered shrub growing extensively along the Atlantic Coast and in the Pacific Northwest, are known variously as broom, broom tops, and Scotch broom. The drug was formerly used in medicine, primarily in the form of a fluid extract, for its diuretic, cathartic, and in large doses, emetic properties. Broom contains up to about 1.5% of the alkaloid sparteine, once employed therapeutically to slow the pulse in cardiac disturbances; this use has now been discontinued in the United States. The plant also contains several other alkaloids and a number of simple amines which contribute to its physiological actions.[1]

In recent years, broom has gained notoriety as a "legal" intoxicant or drug of abuse. Publications aimed at readers in the counterculture[2,3] recommend that the flowers be collected and aged about ten days in a sealed jar. The moldy, dried blossoms thus obtained are then pulverized, rolled in cigaret paper, and smoked like marihuana. One such cigaret is said to produce a feeling of relaxation and euphoria lasting about two hours. Smoking additional amounts, it is claimed, results in deeper relaxation and heightened color awareness without any accompanying visual disturbances or hallucinations.

Although advocates maintain that such use of broom usually does not produce any undesirable effects except a mild headache, the practice has nothing to recommend it. Sparteine, the principal alkaloid in the plant, is contained in the various floral parts in concentrations ranging from 0.01 to 0.22%.[4] It is a volatile compound and unquestionably is present in the smoke inhaled. Sparteine has very pronounced physiological effects, slowing the heart (but not strengthening it) and stimulating uterine contractions. Because of the latter action, the alkaloid was formerly used to induce labor, an application found to be unsafe and now discontinued.

But the greatest potential danger in smoking moldy broom flowers probably lies not in the flowers, but in the fungus infecting them. Studies have shown that almost all samples of illegally obtained marihuana tested were contaminated with pathogenic, inhalable *Aspergillus* species which may sensitize the host.[5] Broom flowers purposely allowed to become moldy would almost certainly be similarly contaminated with such organisms and would thus present an appreciable risk to the user.

Broom does act as a diuretic as a result of having a flavone glycoside, scoparoside, present mostly in the flowers.[6] There are, however, safer and more effective drugs for this and all other actions attributed to the drug. Its employment as a mind-altering agent is potentially dangerous to the user in many ways and is definitely not recommended.

REFERENCES

1. A. Osol and G. E. Farrar, Jr., Eds.: The Dispensatory of the United States of America, 24th Ed. J. B. Lippincott, Philadelphia, 1947, p. 1579.
2. L. A. Young, L. G. Young, M. M. Klein, D. M. Klein, and D. Beyer: Recreational Drugs. Collier Books, New York, 1977, p. 42.
3. A. Gottlieb: Legal Highs. 20th Century Alchemist, Manhattan Beach, Calif., 1973, pp. 6–7.
4. B. T. Cromwell: In Modern Methods of Plant Analysis, Vol. 4, K. Paech and M. V. Tracey, Eds. Springer-Verlag, Berlin, 1955, pp. 460–462.
5. S. L. Kagen, P. G. Sohnle, V. P. Kurup, and J. N. Fink: New England Journal of Medicine 304: 483–484, 1981.
6. E. Steinegger and R. Hänsel: Lehrbuch der Pharmakognosie, 3rd Ed. Springer-Verlag, Berlin, 1972, pp. 291–292.

BUCHU

Helmbold the Buchu King first came to my attention in a lecture I attended as an undergraduate student. My professor told his class how Henry T. Helmbold,[1] a patent medicine producer in New York City, introduced Helmbold's Compound Extract of Buchu in 1847 and advertised it widely as a cure for diabetes, gravel (kidney stones), inflammation of the kidneys, catarrh of the bladder, diseases arising from exposure or imprudence (venereal diseases), nervous diseases, prostration of the system, and the like . . . "from whatever cause originating and whether existing in either sex." As might be anticipated, with a product like that he made a fortune and even aspired to the presidency of the United States!

Buchu consists of the dried leaves of three species of the genus *Barosma* which are given common names based on the leaf shape: *B. betulina* (Thunb.) Bartl. & Wendl., commercially known as short buchu; *B. crenulata* (L.) Hook., called ovate buchu; *B. serratifolia* (Curt.) Willd., known as long buchu. All are obtained from low, white- or pink-flowered shrubs of the family Rutaceae, native to South Africa. Originally utilized as a drug by the Hottentots in that area, the leaves have been used as a household remedy for almost every known affliction. An alcoholic beverage, buchu brandy, is also widely distributed there.[2] The drug used to be official in *The National Formulary* and was rather widely employed as a urinary antiseptic and diuretic. Its use by physicians has been discontinued, but advocates of herbs continue to promote it for the same conditions that Helmbold recommended it more than 130 years ago.

Whatever therapeutic utility buchu may possess is due to its volatile oil, the principal active constituent of which is buchu camphor or diosphenol. This accounts for the incorporation of buchu leaves in a large number of teas still sold in Europe for kidney and bladder conditions.[3] However, its diuretic and especially, its antiseptic properties are relatively mild, and this must be kept in mind if one suffers from a condition that requires an especially effective drug. There is no reason, however, to question the safety of buchu.

REFERENCES

1. H. W. Holcombe: Patent Medicine Tax Stamps. Quarterman Publications, Lawrence, Mass., 1979, pp. 208–213.
2. H. S. Gentry: Economic Botany 15: 326–331, 1961.
3. E. Steinegger and R. Hänsel: Lehrbuch der Pharmakognosie, 3rd Ed. Springer-Verlag, Berlin, 1972, pp. 442–443.

BURDOCK

Burdock consists of the dried, first-year root of *Arctium lappa* L. or *Arctium minus* (Hill) Bernh. The former species is native to Europe but has been naturalized in the United States; the latter is the chief American source of the root. Both are large, coarse biennial herbs with hooked bracts or burs which adhere to clothing or animal fur. *A. lappa* may attain a height of 9 feet, but *A. minus* is limited to about 5 feet. Occasionally, other similar species, such as *Arctium tomentosum* Mill. and *Arctium nemorosum* Lej. & Court., are also utilized.

Recommended primarily as a blood purifier, burdock has also been used to treat various chronic skin conditions, including psoriasis and acne. It is also said to have diuretic and diaphoretic properties.[1] None of these purported effects has been verified by clinical trials, nor have chemical studies of the root revealed the presence of active principles which might account for any such effects. Burdock does contain large amounts of carbohydrate in the form of inulin, together with small amounts of volatile oil, fatty oil, sucrose, resin, tannin, and the like.[2] One interesting study did reveal the presence of some 14 different polyacetylene compounds in the fresh root, 2 of which possessed bacteriostatic and fungistatic properties. However, only traces of them were found in the dried, commercial drug.[3]

One case of poisoning by burdock tea has been reported in the American literature.[4] The patient exhibited all of the symptoms of atropine poisoning, and indeed, the tea was analyzed and found to contain large amounts of that toxic alkaloid. Unfortunately, no evidence was presented to support the contention that the atropine derived from burdock root. In its absence, we can only conclude that another atropine-containing drug, such as belladonna root, was erroneously substituted for burdock.

This conclusion is supported by more recent cases of poisoning with "burdock" tea which occurred in France.[5] There it was possible to examine samples of the burdock root obtained from the wholesaler, who, in turn, had received them from Bulgaria and Yugoslavia. Both were contaminated with atropine-containing belladonna root. These episodes emphasize the hazard of purchasing herbal materials which have not been subjected to proper quality-control procedures.

In spite of its long use as a folkloric remedy, no solid evidence exists that burdock exhibits any useful therapeutic activity. The young leaves may be eaten as greens, and the fresh root may have some antimicrobial properties, but the commercial dried root is lacking in medicinal value.

REFERENCES

1. J. C. Torke: Herbalist 2(4): 124–125, 1977.
2. H. A. Hoppe: Drogenkunde, 8th Ed., Vol. 1. Walter de Gruyter, Berlin, 1975, pp. 102–104.
3. K. E. Schulte, G. Rücker, and R. Boehme: Arzneimittel-Forschung 17: 829–833, 1967.
4. P. D. Bryson, A. S. Watanabe, B. H. Rumack, and R. C. Murphy: Journal of the American Medical Association 239: 2157, 1978.
5. Anon.: Deutsche Apotheker Zeitung 124: 390, 1984.

BUTCHER'S-BROOM

Broom is one of those indefinite common names that tend to make the field of plant-drug nomenclature such a difficult one. The name was originally applied to several plants whose tough stems and rigid leaves made them useful for sweeping up debris. Used without a qualifying adjective, broom refers to the previously discussed *Cytisus scoparius* L., a common roadside plant in the Pacific Northwest, distinguishable by its showy yellow flowers. Spanish broom or gorse (*Spartium junceum* L.) is another yellow-flowered leguminous shrub that flourishes in parts of California. Although both plants have been used in folk medicine, neither is the so-called butcher's-broom which is, so to speak, "sweeping the country" at the present time.

Butcher's-broom, also known as box holly or knee holly, is a fairly common, short evergreen shrub (*Ruscus aculeatus* L.) of the family Liliaceae, native throughout the Mediterranean region from the Azores to Iran. It, too, has a long history of use in herbal medicine. As early as the first century, Dioscorides recommended butcher's-broom as a laxative and diuretic. The 17th century apothecary-astrologer Nicholas Culpeper suggested that a decoction of the root be drunk and a poultice of the berries and leaves applied to facilitate the knitting of broken bones. However, the drug never became popular in either Europe or the United States and, until recently, was seldom mentioned in standard references on drugs.[1]

Then, during the 1950's, French investigators showed that an alcoholic extract of butcher's-broom rhizomes (underground stems) produced vasoconstriction (blood vessel narrowing) in test animals.[2] Further studies identified the active principles as a mixture of steroidal saponins, the two main ones being identified as ruscogenin and neoruscogenin.[3,4] In addition to its vasoconstrictive effects, the extract was demonstrated to have anti-inflammatory properties.

These studies convinced certain European drug manufacturers that butcher's-broom extract is superior to some of the conventional plant remedies, such as extracts of horse chestnut and witch hazel, that are marketed for their supposed beneficial effects on venous circulation. Consequently, they have made extracts of butcher's-broom commercially available in capsule form to treat circulatory problems of the legs, and as an ointment or suppository to relieve the symptoms of hemorrhoids.[5]

Capsules containing 75 mg of butcher's-broom and 2 mg of rosemary oil are now being sold in the United States, mainly through "health food" stores. One such product is being advertised as "a proven European herbal formula—said to improve circulation in the legs," while another is being promoted with the claim that "millions of Europeans report it works wonders—particularly for women who often complain about a 'heavy feeling' in the legs." The ads also state that butcher's-broom is "rare" or "hard-to-find"—which is not true.[6]

While there may be some basis for cautious optimism concerning butcher's-broom as a potentially useful drug, would-be consumers should recognize that manufacturers of butcher's-broom products have never presented proof of safety and efficacy to the Food and Drug Administration and that therapeutic claims for these products are therefore illegal. Moreover, self-diagnosis and self-treatment of circulatory disorders, or any other potentially serious health problem, are certainly inadvisable.

REFERENCES

1. I. Müller: Deutsche Apotheker-Zeitung 113: 1370–1375, 1973.
2. F. Caujolle, P. Mériel, and E. Stanislas: Annales Pharmaceutiques Françaises 11: 109–120, 1953.
3. P. H. List and L. Hörhammer, Eds.: Hagers Handbuch der Pharmazeutischen Praxis, 4th Ed., Vol. 6 B. Springer-Verlag, Berlin, 1979, pp. 200–201.
4. C. Sannie and H. Lapin: Bulletin de la Societe Chimique de France 1957: 1237–1241.
5. R. F. Weiss: Lehrbuch der Phytotherapie, 5th Ed. Hippokrates Verlag, Stuttgart, 1982, pp. 142–143.
6. Better Nutrition 44(1): 17, 1984.

CAFFEINE-CONTAINING PLANTS

"Coffee, though a useful medicine, if drank constantly, will at length induce a decay of health, and hectic fever"
Jesse Torrey
The Moral Instructor, Pt. IV,
Sect. II, Ch. 10

Half-a-dozen caffeine-containing plants are more widely used by mankind, primarily as beverages, than all the other herbal materials put together. These ubiquitous products include:[1]

Coffee — the dried ripe seed of *Coffea arabica* L. or other species of *Coffea* (family Rubiaceae, small evergreen trees or large shrubs cultivated extensively in tropical areas of the world. Deprived of most of the seed coat, the so-called bean is roasted until it becomes dark brown in color and develops a characteristic aroma. Coffee beans contain 1 to 2% of caffeine.

Tea — The prepared leaves and leaf buds of *Camellia sinensis* (L.) O. Kuntze (family Theaceae), a large shrub with evergreen leaves native to eastern Asia and extensively cultivated there. Black tea is prepared by an initial slow drying of the fresh leaves which allows them to begin to ferment. For green tea, a less popular beverage in the United States, the leaves are quickly dried. Because of these different methods of preparation and the many different varieties of the cultivated plant, the average caffeine content of tea ranges widely from about 1 to more than 4%.

Kola (Cola or Kolanuts) — the dried cotyledons (seed leaves) of *Cola nitida* (Vent.) Schott et Endl., or of other species of *Cola* (family Sterculiaceae). The plants are large trees native to West Africa, where much of our commercial supply still comes from, but also cultivated in the West Indies and other tropical lands. Kola contains up to about 3% caffeine.

Cacao (Cocoa) — the roasted seeds of *Theobroma cacao* L. (family Sterculiaceae), a relatively tall tree native to Mexico but now widely cultivated in the tropics. With processing, cacao beans (also called cocoa beans) yield chocolate and all its related products such as breakfast cocoa and cacao (cocoa) butter. Cacao contains between 0.07 and 0.36% caffeine.

Important! Do not confuse cacao or cocoa, which are identical, with coca, the source of cocaine, or with coconut, the palm which yields copra and coconut oil. Cacao (cocoa), coca, and coconut are three entirely different plants, even if the old Marx Brothers' movie with its misspelled title *Cocoanuts* did thoroughly confuse the issue.

Guarana — a dried paste made chiefly from the crushed seed of *Paullinia cupana* H.B.K. (family Sapindaceae), a climbing shrub native to Brazil and Uruguay. The natives of those countries prepare a hot beverage from guarana, and it is employed as an ingredient in a carbonated beverage marketed by the Coca-Cola Company in Brazil. Because of its relatively high caffeine content, ranging from 2.5 to 5% and averaging about 3.5%, guarana has been offered in the U.S. during the last several years under various names, including Zoom, as a "legal" stimulant and cocaine substitute.[2]

Maté — the dried leaves of *Ilex paraguariensis* St. Hil. (family Aquifoliaceae), a small tree or shrub growing wild in Paraguay, Brazil, and other South American countries. Containing up to 2% caffeine, maté or Paraguay tea as it is frequently called, is widely used in South America in the preparation of a tea-like beverage.

In addition to all of these products, which contain caffeine as a natural ingredient, large quantities of the pure stimulant are sold in tablet form and are also utilized as a food additive — particularly in "cola"- or "pepper"-type drinks but also in baked goods, frozen dairy desserts, gelatin puddings and fillings, soft candy, and the like. Some 2 million pounds of caffeine are used annually in this manner in the United States, not including the amounts occurring naturally in various plant materials. In October, 1980, the Food and Drug Administration proposed deletion of caffeine as a food additive from its "generally-recognized-as-safe" (GRAS) list,[3] but as of summer, 1981, no action had been taken, pending further studies. Even if approved, the proposal would limit the use of caffeine only as an additive, not as an ingredient of a natural product.

The important information for the potential consumer of a caffeine-containing plant material is not how much active constituent is present in the crude drug but how much is in the consumed product. Here are approximate amounts of caffeine in some commonly used foods and beverages:[1,2,4,5]

Cup (6 oz) of boiled coffee	100 mg
Cup (6 oz.) of instant coffee	65 mg
Cup (6 oz) of tea	10–50 mg
Bottle or can (12 oz) of cola beverage	50 mg
Cup (6 oz) of breakfast cocoa	13 mg
Bar (1 oz) of milk chocolate	6 mg
Tablet of caffeine (proprietary product)	100–200 mg
Tablet (800 mg) of Zoom (guarana)	60 mg
Cup (6 oz) of maté	25–50 mg

Note that the method of preparation is more important than the caffeine content of the original plant material in determining the concentration in the final product. Tea which may contain 4% caffeine in its leaves seldom has more than 50 mg per cup because it is prepared as an infusion (boiling water is added to the leaves and allowed to cool). Coffee, on the other hand, contains only 1 to 2% caffeine but is usually prepared as a decoction, that is, placed in cold water which is then slowly heated to boiling. Thus, a cup of coffee contains about twice as much caffeine (100 mg) as the same quantity of tea. Of course, the exact amounts vary appreciably because of the different quantities of plant material used by different preparers.

Caffeine is the principal physiologically active constituent in all of these plants, but to alert those concerned about their health, many contain other constituents which may be harmful for long-term usage. For example, there is evidence indicating that the condensed catechin tannin of tea is linked to high rates of esophageal cancer in areas where tea is consumed in large quantities.[6] Incidentally, this effect apparently may be overcome by consuming the tea along with milk, thereby binding the tannin and preventing its deleterious effect. Some evidence linking coffee and cancer of the pancreas has been recorded; this effect, which requires verification, was not tied directly to the content of caffeine.[7]

Caffeine is an effective stimulant of the central nervous system but, especially in large amounts, produces many undesirable side effects — from nervousness and insomnia to rapid and irregular heartbeats, elevated blood sugar and cholesterol levels, excess stomach acid and heartburn. It is definitely a teratogen (produces deformed fetuses) in rats; the FDA has advised practitioners to counsel patients who are or may become pregnant to avoid or limit consumption of foods and drugs containing caffeine.[5]

This is sound advice, for based on our incomplete knowledge of side reactions to caffeine, prudent use seems desirable for all consumers, male and female. The problem is particularly significant in children because the effects of caffeine are related to body weight of the consumer. Nonpregnant adults should probably limit their consumption of caffeine to no more than 250 mg per day.[4] Pregnant women and children should be even more conservative. And moderation in the use of caffeine-containing products should be the watchword for all.

REFERENCES

1. V. E. Tyler, L. R. Brady, and J. E. Robbers: Pharmacognosy, 8th Ed. Lea & Febiger, Philadelphia, 1981, pp. 257 – 260.
2. A. Salsedo: Whole Foods 2(12): 20 – 31, 1979.
3. Federal Register 45(205): 69816 – 69838, Oct. 21, 1980.
4. J. Eddington, Ed.: Update: Cancer Research & Training Newsletter (Purdue University Cancer Center) 5(8): 2, 1980.
5. FDA Drug Bulletin 10(3): 19 – 20, 1980.
6. J. F. Morton: Science 204: 909, 1979.
7. Anon.: Science News 120: 6, 1981.

CALAMUS

Known since biblical times, the aromatic rhizome (underground stem) of *Acorus calamus* L. is commonly referred to as calamus or sweet flag. It has been taken over the centuries as a remedy for various sorts of digestive upsets and colic, especially in children. The plant is a perennial herb of the family Araceae, commonly found in moist habitats such as the banks of ponds or streams and in swamps throughout North America, Europe, and Asia. In appearance, it resembles the iris.

Modern writers on herbs recommend an infusion of the rhizome for fevers and dyspepsia; chewing the rhizome to ease digestion and to clear the voice; and using the powdered material as a substitute for various spices in cooking.[1] Some persons greatly enjoy its flavor. As Brer Rabbit put it, "I done got so now dat I can't eat no chicken 'ceppin she's seasoned up wid calamus root." Calamus is also said to be used as a flavoring agent in a variety of commercial products ranging from tooth powders and tonics to beer and bitters. The volatile oil responsible for the drug's characteristic odor and taste occurs in amounts ranging from 1.5 to more than 3.5%. Unfortunately, feeding studies conducted about 20 years ago established that β-asarone (cis-isoasarone), a major constituent in certain calamus oils, produced malignant tumors in the duodenal region of rats. Since then, use of calamus as a food or food additive has been banned, at least in the United States.[2]

More recent investigations have now shown that there are actually four different drug types of calamus, each originating from a different variety of *Acorus calamus* growing in different geographical areas of the world. Drug type I is found in North America and its oil is isoasarone free. Drug type II is produced in western Europe from plants originating in eastern Europe. Its volatile oil usually contains less than 10% isoasarone. Drug types III and IV are varieties whose volatile oils may contain as much as 96% cis-isoasarone.[3]

Pharmacological tests have now shown that the isoasarone-free oil of drug type 1 has an even more effective spasmolytic (antispasmodic) activity than the isoasarone-rich oil of drug type IV or the isoasarone-poor oil of drug type II.[4] Such results suggest that North American (type I) calamus is an effective herbal remedy for dyspepsia and similar conditions where its antispasmodic effect may produce some relief. The identity of the constituent(s) in the volatile oil that are responsible for this effect remains to be established. Although the absolute safety of type I calamus has yet to be proven by extensive clinical tests, it is at least free of the carcinogenic isoasarone which renders the other drug types unsuitable for medicinal use.

REFERENCES

1. W. H. Hylton, Ed.: The Rodale Herb Book. Rodale Press Book Div. Emmaus, Pa., 1976, pp. 380–381.
2. J. M. Taylor, W. I. Jones, E. C. Hagan, M. A. Gross, D. A. Davis, and E. L. Cook: Toxicology and Applied Pharmacology 10: 405, 1967.
3. K. Keller and E. Stahl: Deutsche Apotheker Zeitung 122: 2463–2466, 1982.
4. K. Keller, K. P. Odenthal, and E. Leng-Peschlow: Planta Medica No. 1: 6–9, 1985.

CALENDULA

The ligulate florets, commonly (but erroneously) referred to as flower petals, of *Calendula officinalis* L. have been used in medicine since the very earliest times. The plant, a member of the family Compositae, is a common cultivated ornamental, also referred to as marigold or garden marigold. During its long history, the drug has been administered internally for a variety of ailments including spasms, fevers, suppressed menstruation, and cancer. Its chief use, however, was as a local application to help heal and prevent infection of lacerated wounds.[1] Modern herbalists recommend it in the form of a tincture, infusion, or ointment to heal a variety of skin conditions ranging from chapped hands to open wounds.[2]

A large number of chemical studies of calendula flowers have been carried out, especially in Europe, without revealing any principles which are unique or even outstanding in their physiological properties. A volatile oil, bitter principles, carotenoids, mucilage, resin, plant acids, various alcohols, saponins and other glycosides, and sterols are all present. Many of the individual constituents in these general groups have been identified.[3]

The carotenoid pigments possess some utility as coloring agents in cosmetics, and the volatile oil is a useful ingredient in perfume, but none of the other known components has medicinal properties which are superior to other available remedies. Calendula is apparently nontoxic, and in an ointment, will be colored sufficiently to delineate a wound or other skin condition where applied. In this regard it is probably as useful as Mercurochrome®. However, one should not expect any particular therapeutic results from its use, other than those provided by the placebo effect.

REFERENCES

1. H. W. Felter and J. U. Lloyd: King's American Dispensatory, 18th Ed., Vol. 1. The Ohio Valley Co., Cincinnati, 1898, pp. 401–403.
2. D. D. Buchman: Herbalist 2(3): 80–84, 1977.
3. P. H. List and L. Hörhammer, Eds.: Hagers Handbuch der Pharmazeutischen Praxis, 4th Ed., Vol. 3. Springer-Verlag, Berlin, 1972, pp. 603–608.

CANAIGRE

Canaigre, the root of *Rumex hymenosepalus* Torr., has been marketed recently under such coined names of modern vintage as wild red American ginseng and wild red desert ginseng. The plant, a member of the family Polygonaceae native to the deserts of the southwestern United States and Mexico, actually bears no relationship either botanically or in its active principles to ginseng which belongs to an entirely different family, the Araliaceae.

Current promotional literature on canaigre indicates that the drug was recommended in old herbals for a large number of maladies ranging from lack of vitality to leprosy.[1] Unfortunately, the authors of such statements somehow fail to include references, and an inspection of herbal literature does not substantiate this claim. For example, J. M. Nickell's comprehensive listing of some 2500 botanical remedies in 1911 omits the plant entirely.[2] *King's American Dispensatory* (1900), a comprehensive eclectic compendium devoting 2172 closely written pages to plant remedies, dedicates eight lines of fine print to canaigre, stating that because of its high tannin content, it was used for tanning and dyeing by the Indians.[3] Not a single word therein notes any medicinal use. Voelcker, however, mentions in 1876 that the natives of Mexico used the root as an astringent.[4]

It is obvious that the attempt to promote canaigre as a kind of American ginseng is a recent deceptive practice, probably due to the high prices commanded by the ginseng of today. Canaigre does not contain any of the active panaxoside-like saponin glycosides responsible for ginseng's physiological activities. It does contain 18 to 25% or more of tannin and smaller amounts of anthraquinones, as well as other constituents such as starch and resin.[5]

Recognizing this attempt to substitute a relatively common, essentially worthless plant for a more valuable commodity, the Herb Trade Association adopted a policy statement in 1979[6] "that any herb products consisting in whole or part of *Rumex hymenosepalus* should not be labeled as containing 'ginseng.'" Nevertheless, canaigre continues to be advertised by at least one marketer[7] as "a natural alternative to ginseng."

Canaigre may thus be a useful material for tanning leather and dyeing wool, but it has no place in therapeutics. Indeed, because of its high tannin content, the root may have considerable carcinogenic potential. Rational people will avoid using it or any capsules or extracts prepared from it.

> "You can't make a silk purse out of a sow's ear."
> Jonathan Swift
> *Polite Conversation*

REFERENCES

1. D. L. Poulson: Herbalist 3(1): 16–17, 1978.
2. J. M. Nickell: J. M. Nickell's Botanical Ready Reference, Murray & Nickell Mfg. Co., Chicago, 1911.
3. H. W. Felter and J. U. Lloyd: King's American Dispensatory, 18th Ed., Vol. 2 The Ohio Valley Company, Cincinnati, 1900, p. 1685.
4. R. F. G. Voelcker: American Journal of Pharmacy 48: 49–51, 1876.
5. C. Wehmer: Die Pflanzenstoffe, 2nd Ed., Vol. 1. Verlag von Gustav Fischer, Jena, 1929, p. 275.
6. Herb Trade Association: Policy Statement #1 — Canaigre, May, 1979.
7. Territorial Mfg. & Dist., Inc.: Whole Foods 3(1): 24, 1980.

CAPSICUM

Capsicum, cayenne pepper or chili pepper, is also referred to merely as red pepper. It consists of the dried ripe fruit of *Capsicum frutescens* L., *Capsicum annuum* L., or a large number of hybrids or varieties of these species of the family Solanaceae. For centuries, these plants have been highly valued as spices, and the extensive cultivation carried out over that period of time has resulted in peppers widely differing from one another in size, shape, and pungency. The labeling of commercial samples is really meaningful only if the variety is specifically designated.[1]

Applied externally, capsicum is a rubifacient, that is, an agent that reddens the skin, thereby producing a counterirritant effect. Internally, it is valued as a stomachic, carminative, and gastrointestional stimulant.[2] All of these activities depend upon the presence in capsicum of a compound known as capsaicin which, together with two closely related principles, is responsible for the pungency of the fruit. In addition, capsicum serves as a relatively good source of vitamin C.

As is the case with so many herbs, the modest but real utility of capsicum tends to be obscured by the exaggerated claims made for it by over-enthusiastic advocates. It has been reported that people in Mexico and Hungary have a low incidence of atherosclerosis and relatively few heart attacks because they eat large amounts of capsicum.[3] This statement is without any scientific basis.

As an external counterirritant, capsicum is quite effective. Its action is fairly long lasting, and it does not blister the skin.[4] However, care must be taken not to get it into the eye, or extreme discomfort may result. Capsicum-containing mixtures intended to be placed in the stockings to keep the feet warm on cold days are currently marketed. While they may be modestly effective, the temporary warmth they provide is offset by the risk that, when used by children, some of the pepper may accidentally get into their eyes, resulting in considerable pain.

Persons who pick or otherwise handle quantities of hot peppers recognize that the pungent principle capsaicin is essentially insoluble in cold water and only slightly soluble in hot water. Traces remaining on the hands may be transferred inadvertently to sensitive mucous membranes even several hours after contact. The capsaicin may be removed from the affected part of the anatomy by bathing in vinegar, but, of course, this should not be applied in or around the eye.[5]

Internally, there are great individual variations in the sensitivity of persons to capsicum. The quantity that would prove to be a useful stomachic or digestive aid in one person might be very irritating, even upsetting, to another. Caution in the use of this irritating product is certainly advisable.

REFERENCES

1. V. E. Tyler, L. R. Brady, and J. E. Robbers: Pharmacognosy, 8th Ed. Lea & Febiger, Philadelphia, 1981, pp. 155–156.
2. R. A. Locock: Canadian Pharmaceutical Journal 118: 516–519, 1985.
3. M. Pahlow: Deutsche Apotheker Zeitung 126: 794–795, 1986.
4. T. Sollmann: A Manual of Pharmacology, 7th Ed. W. B. Saunders Company, Philadelphia, 1948, p. 137.
5. T. P. Vogl: New England Journal of Medicine 306: 178, 1982.

CATNIP

"Cats are said to be very fond of it."

It seems strange that the relationship between cats and catnip should have been regarded with such skepticism by an authority on drugs of such stature as *The United States Dispensatory*, 2nd Edition, published in 1834. Not until the 17th Edition, published in 1896, was the sentence changed to:

"Cats are very fond of it . . . ."

Apparently, after more than 60 years, one of the authors of this respected reference finally observed the not uncommon interaction between a cat and the plant whose various names, catnip, catnep, and cat mint, all suggest fairly close affinity.

The dried leaves and flowering tops of the common, wayside, perennial plant *Nepeta cataria* L. contain a volatile oil which is indeed extremely attractive to cats, causing them to cavort playfully while attempting to saturate their entire bodies with the plant's distinctive aroma. Catnip was once rather widely used in human medicine, primarily as a carminative or digestive aid and as a tonic. The hot tea taken at bedtime has also been recommended as a sleep aid. But Gibbons gives his opinion, and it is probably factual, that most catnip tea enthusiasts drink it simply because they like the taste of this pleasant beverage.[1]

In more recent times, catnip has been promoted by certain members of the counterculture as a psychedelic drug, said to produce a sense of well-being or euphoria when smoked like tobacco or marihuana. Unfortunately, the physicians who first described this use in an article in *The Journal of the American Medical Association* confused the identity of the drug, erroneously labeling a drawing of a marihuana plant as catnip and vice versa.[2] Some 1,612 letters pointing out this error were received by the editor, and one writer commented: "Perhaps one reason for his patients getting high on catnip is their lack of botanical knowledge."[3]

It is an unfortunate fact that once an erroneous statement has appeared in print, it is almost impossible to eradicate it. Catnip now is listed in practically all books devoted to drugs of abuse as a mild intoxicant. One of the more cautious of these[4] begins its discussion of the plant with the statement, "Does it or doesn't it?" The book then goes on to indicate that a debate has raged for years among potheads as to whether one can actually get "high" by using catnip. Any drug whose mind-altering effects are as questionable as this one is scarcely worth considering for that purpose. Yet the plant does contain a volatile oil, the odor of which causes a series of characteristic stimulatory responses in *cats*. The active principle responsible for these effects is a compound designated *cis-trans*-nepetalactone; it is a major component, constituting 70 to 99% of the volatile oil. Interestingly, it produces its effects in cats only when it is smelled, not when it is administered orally.[5] However, nepetalactone is somewhat similar in its chemical structure to the valepotriates, the sedative principles of valerian.[6] Thus, there just may be some basis in fact for the cup of hot catnip tea taken at bedtime to insure a good night's sleep. Besides, it's relatively inexpensive, it tastes good, and no harmful effects from using it have been reported. What more can one ask of a beverage?

REFERENCES

1. E. Gibbons: Stalking the Healthful Herbs, Field Guide Ed. David McKay Co., New York, 1970. p. 84.
2. B. Jackson and A. Reed: Journal of the American Medical Association 207: 1349–1350, 1969.
3. J. Poundstone: *Ibid*. 208: 360, 1969.
4. L. A. Young, L. G. Young, M. M. Klein, D. M. Klein, and D. Beyer: Recreational Drugs. Collier Books, New York, 1977, p. 52.
5. G. R. Waller, G. H. Price, and E. D. Mitchell: Science 164: 1281–1282, 1969.
6. M. Kuklinski: Deutsche Apotheker-Zeitung 109: 114, 1969.

THE CHAMOMILES AND YARROW

Three plants, closely related botanically and chemically, have long enjoyed great popularity as folk remedies useful in treating digestive disorders, cramps, various skin conditions and minor infectious ailments. All three are members of the Compositae or daisy family and all yield a blue-colored volatile oil. Most volatile oils are local irritants, but those which contain quantities of the intensely blue compound chamazulene, together with other active ingredients, have anti-inflammatory properties.

Two of the plants are known as chamomile. They consist of the flowerheads of *Matricaria chamomilla* L., known as German or Hungarian Chamomile, and *Anthemis nobilis* L., also called Roman or English chamomile. The plants are similar in appearance, but the German variety is an erect annual while Roman chamomile is a nearly prostrate perennial. Both possess a distinct apple-like fragrance and flavor. The third plant consists of the flowering herb (entire overground plant) of *Achillea millefolium* L., commonly called yarrow. Because of their popularity as household medicines, all of the plants, but especially the chamomiles, are extensively cultivated. Their chemical constituents have also been subject to detailed study. Interestingly, with the exception of the common denominator, chamazulene, the composition of the plants and their contained volatile oils is quite varied.[1]

Of the trio, German chamomile (the Germans refer to it as genuine chamomile) has been the most extensively investigated from the pharmacological and chemical viewpoints. It is used everywhere in Europe almost as a panacea, but basically as a carminative (aids digestion), an anti-inflammatory for various afflictions of the skin and mucous membranes, as an antispasmodic primarily for treating menstrual cramps, and as an anti-infective for all kinds of minor illnesses. Extracts of the plant or its volatile oil are used in the form of ointments, lotions, vapor baths, inhalations, and the like, all intended for local application. Internally, the drug is taken as a strong tea.

Many believe that chamomile will cure almost anything; indeed, the Germans have a phrase for it, *alles zutraut*, meaning "capable of anything." As a popular remedy, it may be thought of as the European counterpart of ginseng. Some think that both patients and physicians would be better off if chamomile were even more widely used:

"How the Doctor's brow should smile
Crown'd with wreaths of camomile."
Thomas Moore
Wreaths for the Ministers

Chamazulene and a terpene derivative designed (-)-α-bisabolol are primarily responsible for the anti-inflammatory activity of German chamomile. Both are found in the volatile oil, the latter as a major constituent (up to 50%). Studies have shown that (-)-α-bisabolol also protects against peptic ulcer and exhibits antibacterial and antifungal properties. These volatile oil constituents and others, including bisabololoxides A and B and the spiroethers, also contribute to the musculotropic spasmolytic (relaxes smooth muscle) activity of chamomile. However, this property is enhanced by certain non-volatile constituents found in the plant. Specifically, various flavones, especially apigenin, luteolin, patuletin, and quercitin as well as several coumarin derivatives, are active antispasmodics. It is clear that the therapeutic value of chamomile does not rest on a single constituent but on a complex mixture of chemically different compounds.[2]

Since much of the value of the plant lies in its volatile oil, it is unfortunate that even a strong tea, properly prepared in a covered vessel and steeped for a long time, contains only about 10–15% of the volatile oil originally present in the plant material.[3] Whole extracts of the drug or preparations containing quantities of the volatile oil are certainly more effective but are not generally marketed in the United States. Nevertheless, Farnsworth and Morgan[4] believe that when the tea is used over a long period, beneficial effects may accumulate. This belief is supported by the long-time usage of chamomile as a valued folk remedy in Europe and by its increasing popularity in this country.

However, we must conclude these generally favorable comments on the chamomiles and yarrow with a word of caution. Because all three drugs include the flower-heads which contain pollen, tea made from any of them may cause contact dermatitis, anaphylaxis, or other hypersensitivity reactions in allergic individuals.[5] These reactions are, however, relatively infrequent. A survey of the worldwide literature revealed only about 50 reports of allergies resulting from the use of chamomile between the years 1887 and 1982.[6] Of these, only 5 were attributed to *Matricaria chamomilla* (German chamomile). Most of the others were caused by *Anthemis* species (Roman chamomile). The relative infrequency of chamomile hypersensitivity should certainly not deter normal persons from consuming it, if they so desire. However, persons known to be allergic to ragweed, asters, chrysanthemums, or other members of the family Compositae should be cautious about drinking tea prepared from the chamomiles or yarrow.

REFERENCES

1. E. Steinegger and R. Hänsel: Lehrbuch der Pharmakognosie, 3rd Ed. Springer-Verlag, Berlin, 1972, pp. 415–417, 506.
2. O. Isaac: Deutsche Apotheker Zeitung 120: 567–570, 1980.
3. V. E. Tyler, L. R. Brady, and J. E. Robbers: Pharmacognosy, 8th Ed. Lea & Febiger, Philadelphia, 1981, pp. 476–477.
4. N. R. Farnsworth and B. M. Morgan: Journal of the American Medical Association 221: 410, 1972.
5. M. Abramowicz, Ed.: Medical Letter on Drugs and Therapeutics 21(7): 30, 1979.
6. B. M. Hausen, E. Busker, and R. Carle: Planta Medica 50: 229–234, 1984.

CHAPARRAL

Chaparral refers broadly to any dense thicket of shrubs or dwarf trees. More specifically, in recent herbal literature it designates the leaflets of *Larrea tridentata* (DC.) Coville, a name considered by modern authors to be synonymous with *Larrea divaricata* Cav. This strong-scented, olive-green bush of the family Zygophyllaceae is the dominant shrub in the desert regions of the southwestern United States and Mexico. Better known common names of the plant are creosote bush and greasewood.

An aqueous extract of the leaves and twigs, so-called chaparral tea, is an old Indian remedy and has been used for a wide variety of ailments including arthritis, cancer, venereal disease, tuberculosis, bowel cramps, rheumatism and colds. It is said to possess analgesic, expectorant, emetic, diuretic, and anti-inflammatory properties. One of its more unusual applications is that of a hair tonic.[1] Another is its purported property of "taking the residue of LSD out of the system . . . so you will have no recurrences of hallucinations."[2]

As might be expected, most of the attention focused on chaparral tea in recent years has concerned its use, and that of its principal ingredient, nordihydroguaiaretic acid (NDGA), as an anticancer agent. NDGA is a potent antioxidant, especially for fats and oils. As such, it was once thought to be potentially useful in the treatment of cancer. Early studies in rats did indicate that NDGA exerted an inhibitory effect on some tumor cells, but follow-up studies with the tea in human beings have to date proved equivocal.[3] Besides, NDGA possesses considerable toxicity; long-term feeding studies in rats induced lesions in the mesenteric lymph nodes and kidneys. As a result, the compound was removed from the FDA's "generally recognized as safe" (GRAS) list in 1968. However, it must be noted that the U.S. Department of Agriculture, which controls the use of antioxidants in lard and animal shortenings, still permits NDGA to be added to them.

Nevertheless, chaparral possesses no proven medicinal value, and since its principal ingredient is considered by the FDA to be unsafe for human consumption, we cannot recommend the use of this plant for therapeutic purposes.

Mosquitoes, however, have come to view chaparral and its contained NDGA quite differently. When fed the latter compound, the mosquito *Aedes aegypti* lengthened its average lifespan from 29 to 45 days.[5] Wouldn't it be nice if NDGA had the same effect on human beings? Researchers, get busy!

REFERENCES

1. B. N. Timmerman: Creosote Bush: Biology and Chemistry of Larrea In New World Deserts, T. J. Mabry, J. H. Hunziker, and D. R. DiFeo, Jr., Eds. Dowden, Hutchinson & Ross, Stroudsburg, Pa., 1977, pp. 252–256.
2. N. Baird: Herbalist 3(6): 6–8, 1978.
3. D. Mowrey: *Ibid.* 3(6): 28–30, 1978.
4. R. Winter: A Consumer's Dictionary of Food Additives, Rev. Ed. Crown Publishers, Inc., New York, 1984, p. 176.
5. S. Boxer, Ed.: Discover 8(1): 13–14, 1987.

CHICKWEED

Despite the fact that it is prominently listed in almost every catalog of herbs currently available and also that many writers describe it as a valuable herb (Gibbons,[1] for example, devotes six pages to the "useful" chickweed), I can think of no good reason to allow space to this worthless weed. Nevertheless, because people are apt to be misled by uncritical advocates of the medicinal use of chickweed, it is probably worthwhile to give it brief consideration.

Chickweed consists of the leaves and stems of *Stellaria media* (L.) Cyr. of the family Caryophyllaceae, a low-growing or procumbent annual herb with small, white, star-shaped flowers. It is found throughout the world, having become a serious weed in many areas. Modern herbal advocates recommend chickweed for a large number of maladies ranging from constipation to hydrophobia.[2] A poultice of the plant is to be applied locally for every type of skin disease, including boils, abscesses, and ulcers. Taken internally, chickweed is supposed to be useful in curing bronchial asthma, stomach and bowel problems, blood disorders, lung disease, and obesity.

The plant is edible and makes tasty salads or cooked greens. Like many other green leafy vegetables, it contains some vitamin C (0.1 to 0.15%), accounting for its reputation as a cure for scurvy. Other constituents include the flavonoid glycoside rutin and various plant acids, esters, and alcohols.[3] Although there is an extensive scientific literature devoted to chickweed, there is no indication in it that any of the plant's constituents possess pronounced therapeutic value; indeed, most writings concern various methods of controlling this pesky weed.

Let's not waste any more time and space on the imagined medicinal value of this ineffective herb.

REFERENCES

1. E. Gibbons: Stalking the Healthful Herbs, Field Guide Ed. David McKay Company, New York, 1970, pp. 175–179.
2. W. Smith: Wonders in Weeds. Health Science Press, Bradford, England, 1977, pp. 48–50.
3. P. H. List and L. Hörhammer, Eds.: Hagers Handbuch der Pharmazeutischen Praxis 4th Ed., Vol. 6B. Springer-Verlag, Berlin, 1979, pp. 526–527.

CHICORY

Like many Americans, I first tasted chicory in New Orleans. The café au lait served there on the patio of the Café du Monde Coffee Stand overlooking Jackson Square and the Mississippi River levee is a mixture of strong chicory coffee and hot milk, about half and half. Accompanied by crisp, hot beignets dusted with powdered sugar, the beverage provides a delightful experience. To my taste, it was bitter but mellow, two terms I previously thought contradictory!

Chicory or succory, known botanically as *Cichorium intybus* L., is a perennial member of the daisy family (Compositae), native to Europe but now found growing wild along roadsides and in neglected fields throughout North America. Attaining a height of 3 to 5 feet or more, it is conspicuous for its attractive azure-blue flowers. The plant has been grown in large quantities in Europe for many years in order to supply the demands of the beverage industry for roasted chicory root as a coffee additive or substitute. There is also a demand for the leaves which are used in salads and as greens. As a consequence, there exist many cultivated varieties which differ primarily in the size and texture of their roots and leaves.[1]

In folk medicine, chicory root is valued primarily as a mild non-irritating tonic with associated diuretic and, particularly, laxative effects.[2] It is said to protect the liver from and act as a counterstimulant to the effects of excessive coffee drinking.[3] Chicory root is valued in Egypt as a folk remedy for tachycardia (rapid heartbeat). The bruised leaves are considered to make a good poultice and are applied locally for the relief of swellings and inflammations. In addition, they are valued as a leafy green vegetable.

A rather large number of chemical constituents have been identified in chicory root, but none is especially physiologically active. They include 11 to 15% (up to 58% in cultivated plants) of the polysaccharide inulin, 10 to 22% of fructose, the bitter principles lactucin and lactucopicrin, tannin, both a fatty and a volatile oil, and small amounts of several other compounds.[4] From the culinary viewpoint, the inulin is particularly interesting. On roasting, it is converted to oxymethylfurfurol, a compound with a coffee-like aroma.

For more than 40 years, a scientific report has existed in the literature that lactucin and, to a lesser extent, lactucopicrin produce a sedative effect on the central nervous system and are capable of antagonizing the stimulant properties of caffeine beverages.[5] This work carried out in rabbits and mice may explain some of the old tales about chicory countering the undesirable "nervous" effects of coffee. However, much more study is needed, including quantitative measurements of the bitter principles in various varieties of the root, before a definite conclusion can be reached.

A more recent investigation by Egyptian scientists studying the folkloric reputation of chicory as a drug useful in treating tachycardia apparently showed the presence of a digitalis-like principle in both the dried and roasted root which decreased the rate and amplitude of the heartbeat.[6] Its effects were demonstrated in the toad heart, and the activity in different samples, which incidentally varied greatly, was measured by the Baljet reaction, a color test for cardioactive glycosides. The active principle was not isolated, and the significance of this finding is very difficult to assess without additional information.

Since chicory has been consumed in such large quantities by so many people for so many years without any reported untoward effects, it is difficult to believe that it has the ability to produce any pronounced physiological or therapeutic actions in human beings. The conclusion is inevitable. Chicory is certainly as safe and has much less effect on the nervous system and the heart than the caffeine-rich coffee with which it is usually mixed. I think it's still all right to patronize the Café du Monde.

REFERENCES

1. M. Stuart, Ed.: The Encyclopedia of Herbs and Herbalism. Grosset & Dunlap, New York, 1979, p. 173.
2. R. C. Wren and R. W. Wren: Potter's New Cyclopaedia of Botanical Drugs and Preparations, New Ed. Health Science Press, Hengiscote, England, 1975, p. 80.
3. M. Grieve: A Modern Herbal, Vol. 1. Dover Publications, New York, 1971, pp. 197–199.
4. P. H. List and L. Hörhammer, Eds.: Hagers Handbuch der Pharmazeutischen Praxis, 4th Ed., Vol. 4. Springer-Verlag, Berlin, 1973, pp. 3–5.
5. A. W. Forst: Naunyn-Schmiedebergs Archiv für experimentelle Pathologie und Pharmakologie 195: 1–25, 1940.
6. S. I. Balboa, A. Y. Zaki, S. M. Abdel-Wahab, E. S. M. El-Denshary, and M. Motazz-Bellah: Planta Medica 24: 133–144, 1973.

COLTSFOOT

Coltsfoot, the dried leaves and/or flowerheads of *Tussilago farfara* L., is one of those plants whose botanical name reflects its medicinal application. *Tussilago* derives from the Latin *tussis* meaning cough, and the plant has long been used to treat that affliction. This member of the family Compositae is a low, perennial, woolly herb which early in the spring produces a flowering stem with a single terminal yellow flower-head. After the flower stem dies down, the hoof-shaped leaves appear. The plant is native to Europe but grows widely in moist, sandy places in the northeastern and north central United States and southern Canada.[1] Since the flowers and leaves appear at different times, they are collected and marketed separately.

Over the years, coltsfoot has been a very popular folk remedy for coughs and bronchial congestion. Both the leaves and blossoms are ingredients in a large number of proprietary tea mixtures which are marketed in Europe for treating these conditions.[2] Gibbons has given recipes for preparing coltsfoot cough drops, coltsfoot cough syrup, and coltsfoot tea.[3] He also provided a formula for an herbal smoking mixture, like British Herb Tobacco, which consists principally of coltsfoot and is smoked to "cure coughs and wheezes." Since the principal active ingredient in the plant is a throat-soothing mucilage, smoking coltsfoot is certainly not rational therapy. The mucilage would be destroyed by burning, and the effect of smoke on already irritated mucous membranes would be increased irritation. Inhaling the vapors from coltsfoot leaves placed in a pan of simmering water, as suggested by Bricklin,[4] is again without value. The useful mucilage is not volatile and would not reach the affected tissues.

A scientific study carried out in Japan recently has revealed some rather disturbing information about coltsfoot.[5] The investigators analyzed dried young flowers because they are the parts widely used as an herbal remedy in Japan. They found the hepatotoxic (poisonous to the liver), pyrrolizidine alkaloid senkirkine to be present in relatively small amounts (0.015%). When rats were fed diets containing various amounts of coltsfoot, those which received high concentrations (greater than 4%) developed cancerous tumors of the liver. The scientists concluded that "it is evident that the young, preblooming flowers of coltsfoot are carcinogenic, showing a high incidence of hemangioendothelial sarcoma of the liver (8/12, 66.6%)."

For some time it was hoped that the rest of the plant might be devoid of pyrrolizidine alkaloids. However, a subsequent investigation of coltsfoot leaves showed senkirkine to be present in them as well.[6]

People suffering from throat irritations can no longer consider coltsfoot preparations appropriate therapy. Neither the flowers nor the leaves can safely be used for medicinal purposes. If readers want an herbal demulcent (soothing agent), they should consider a drug such as slippery elm bark or marsh mallow root, both of which long held official status in The United States Pharmacopeia (U.S.P.) and The National Formulary.[7]

REFERENCES

1. H. W. Youngken: Textbook of Pharmacognosy, 6th Ed. The Blakiston Company, Philadelphia, 1948, pp. 888–889.
2. P. H. List and L. Hörhammer, Eds.: Hagers Handbuch der Pharmazeutischen Praxis, 4th Ed., Vol. 6C. Springer-Verlag, Berlin, 1979, pp. 324–329.
3. E. Gibbons: Stalking the Healthful Herbs, Field Guide Ed. David McKay Company, New York, 1970, pp. 29–33.
4. M. Bricklin: The Practical Encyclopedia of Natural Healing. Rodale Press, Emmaus, Pa., 1976, p. 248.
5. I. Hirono, H. Mori, and C. C. J. Culvenor: Gann 67: 125–129, 1976.
6. L. W. Smith and C. C. J. Culvenor: Journal of Natural Products (Lloydia) 44: 129–152, 1981.
7. E. P. Claus and V. E. Tyler, Jr.: Pharmacognosy, 5th Ed. Lea & Febiger, Philadelphia, 1965, p. 85.

COMFREY

Seldom does one encounter the degree of enthusiasm about anything which the modern herbalists display for comfrey, the rhizome and roots as well as the leaves of *Symphytum officinale* L. (family Boraginaceae). These writers emphasize the plant's nearly universal healing properties as well as its safety in such statements as: ". . . the first of all the 'wonder drugs'"[1]; ". . . one of the most important therapeutic agents ever discovered by man"[2]; ". . . a most unusual plant with many preventive and curative properties"[3]; ". . . has a healing and soothing effect upon every organ it contracts"[4]; ". . . an ideal herb for making home remedies for use by amateur herbalists . . . nonpoisonous and completely harmless. . . ."[5]; ". . . a safe and harmless remedy"[6]; "Toxicity is unlikely even after ingestion of moderately large quantities. . . ."[7] The list of quotations could go on and on, but the hyperbole remains the same.

Basically, comfrey is used in folk medicine in the form of an externally applied poultice for healing wounds. It is also taken internally as a tea or blended plant extract (so-called green drink) to heal stomach ulcers and to act as a "blood purifier."[8] Less-restrained advocates preach its virtue in treating cuts and wounds, burns, respiratory ailments of the lungs and bronchial passages, and ulcers of the bowels, stomach, liver, and gallbladder.[2] It is even said to facilitate the healing of broken bones, but this almost certainly comes from a misunderstanding of one of the common names of the plant, knitbone. It may have once been used to reduce the swelling and inflammation around a broken bone, but not to heal the bone itself.

Whatever healing properties comfrey may have are probably caused by its content of allantoin, an agent which promotes cell proliferation. Quantities of tannin and mucilage are also present. The underground parts contain 0.6 to 0.7% allantoin and 4 to 6.5% tannin; the leaves are poorer in allantoin, containing only about 1.3%, but richer in tannin, 8–9%. Large amounts of mucilage are present in both roots and leaves.[9] Much has been made of the vitamin B_{12} content of comfrey, but compared to the more customary natural source, liver, the concentration in the plant is not especially high.[1]

Although comfrey is presently one of the most common herbs sold to the American public, there is reason to believe that using it internally is definitely hazardous to the health. Common comfrey contains several pyrrolizidine alkaloids, of which echimidine and symphytine have been definitely identified.[10] Both root and leaf of this plant have been shown to be carcinogenic in rats when fed in concentrations of as little as 0.5% and 8% of their diet, respectively.[11] Eight pyrrolizidine alkaloids of the hepatotoxic type have been identified in the closely related Russian comfrey, *Symphytum* × *uplandicum* Nym. Tests showed that these combined alkaloids caused chronic hepatotoxicity in rats and raised concern regarding human consumption of the plant.[12]

Such concerns about the toxicity of comfrey have apparently been justified by a recent clinical report. Typical symptoms of chronic pyrrolizidine-alkaloid intoxication were observed in a 49-year-old woman who consumed both tea and capsules containing comfrey.[13] Serious liver damage, known technically as Budd-Chiari syndrome, resulted from a daily intake of one quart of comfrey-containing herbal tea for a period of six months and of six comfrey-pepsin capsules for four months prior to hospitalization. The paucity of previous reports of comfrey toxicity in humans, in spite of many years of general use as a herbal remedy, should not therefore be thought of as an indicator of safety of the product. Instead, such infrequency of recognized toxicity appears to be the result of the slowly cumulative effects of the toxic constituents which delay overt damage and may prevent direct association of it, when it is finally observed, with the plant material. In fairness, however, it must be noted that at least some samples of common comfrey appear to be devoid of pyrrolizidine alkaloids.[14] Such variation among different specimens and the reasons for it require further study.

In the meantime, one comprehensive book on comfrey[1] bears a label on its back cover reminiscent of the required health-hazard warning on cigaret packages. This one reads, in part, ". . . we say that you or your animals should not eat, drink, or take comfrey raw, cooked, flour, tablets, or tea. There is a risk in internal use." It's too bad every comfrey plant which has not been analyzed and found to be free of carcinogenic pyrrolizidine alkaloids — as well as all packages of the drug sold in "health food" stores, most of which contain plant material of undetermined origin — are not similarly labeled.

REFERENCES

1. L. D. Hills: Comfrey. Universe Books, New York, 1976.

2. J. R. Christopher: Herbalist 1(5): 161–166, 1976.
3. G. J. Binding: About Comfrey. Thorsons Publishers Ltd., Welling-borough, England, 1974, p. 23.
4. M. Tierra: The Way of Herbs. Unity Press, Santa Cruz, Calif., 1980. p. 89.
5. E. Gibbons: Stalking the Useful Herbs, Field Guide Ed. David McKay Company, New York, 1970, p. 58.
6. W. Smith: Wonders in Weeds. Health Science Press, Bradford, England, 1977, p. 57.
7. D. G. Spoerke, Jr.: Herbal Medications, Woodbridge Press Publishing Co., Santa Barbara, Calif., 1980, p. 62
8. T. Messina: Herbalist New Health 6(3): 28–29, 1981.
9. P. H. List and L. Hörhammer, Eds.: Hagers Handbuch der Pharmazeutischen Praxis, 4th Ed., Vol. 5B. Springer-Verlag, Berlin, 1979, pp. 706–710.
10. T. Furuya and K. Araki: Chemical and Pharmaceutical Bulletin 16: 2512–2516, 1968.
11. I. Hirono, H. Mori, and M. Haga: Journal of the National Cancer Institute 61:865–869,1978.
12. C. C. J. Culvenor, M. Clarke, J. A. Edgar, J. L. Frahn, M. V. Jago, J. E. Peterson, and L. W. Smith: Experientia 36: 377–379, 1980.
13. P. M. Ridker, S. Ohkuma, W. V. McDermott, C. Trey, and R. J. Huxtable: Gastroenterology 88: 1050–1054, 1985.
14. N. R. Farnsworth: Report of the Botanical Codex Committee American Society of Pharmacognosy, July 30–Aug. 3, 1979, West Lafayette, Ind. (unpublished).

Note added during publication.

An excellent review on comfrey has recently appeared (D.V.C. Awang: Canadian Pharmaceutical Journal 120: 100-104, 1987). In it, and in personal correspondence, Dr. Awang notes several important points. There has been a glaring lack of attention to proper botanical identification of *Symphytum* species by many herbal investigators. *S. officinale* does not (as previously noted) contain echimidine. Instead, that toxic alkaloid is found in *S. asperum* Lepech. (prickly comfrey) and its hybrid *S. x uplandicum*. Further, all comfrey species investigated have been found to contain pyrrolizidine alkaloids. The report that some specimens of common comfrey are free of such alkaloids resulted from a laboratory error.

CUCURBITA

Seeds of several species of the genus *Cucurbita* have long enjoyed a considerable reputation as teniafuges (agents which paralyze and expel intestinal worms). Chief among these are pumpkin seeds or pepo, obtained from *C. pepo* L., but the seeds of the autumn squash (*C. maxima Duchesne*) and of the Canada pumpkin or crookneck squash [*C. moschata* (Duchesne) Poir.] have similar properties.[1] All are large edible fruits produced by herbaceous, running (vinelike) plants of the family Cucurbitaceae. Numerous cultivated varieties exist.

When used as a teniafuge or anthelmintic, cucurbita seeds are ordinarily administered in the form of the ground seeds themselves, as an infusion (tea), or as an emulsion made by beating the seeds with powdered sugar and milk or water. Usually three divided doses are given, representing a total weight of seeds ranging from 60 to as much as 500 grams. Such treatment is said to be effective in expelling both tapeworms and roundworms.[2] Another traditional use of the seeds is in the prevention and treatment of chronic prostatic hypertrophy (enlargement of the prostate gland) in males. A handful of the seeds eaten daily is supposed to be a very popular remedy for this condition in Bulgaria, Turkey, and the Ukraine.[3]

Cucurbitin, an unusual amino acid identified chemically as (-)-3-amino-3-carboxypyrrolidine, is the active principle responsible for the anthelmintic (worm-expelling) effects of the drug. It occurs only in the seeds of *Cucurbita* species, but its concentration is quite variable even in seeds of the same species. This variability probably accounts for reports in the literature that cucurbita seeds are either unreliable or ineffective as a teniafuge. One study showed the concentration of cucurbitin in different samples of *C. pepo* ranged from 1.66 to 6.63%, in *C. maxima* from 5.29 to 19.37%, and in *C. moschata* from 3.98 to 8.44%.[4]

Identifying the principle(s) responsible for any beneficial effects on the prostate gland is not so straightforward. The fatty oil contained in cucurbita seeds in amounts approaching 50% is an efficient diuretic,[2] so the increased urine flow it produces may give an illusory sense of reduction of prostatic swelling or hypertrophy. Administration of unsaturated fatty acids is thought by some to be beneficial in the treatment of prostate problems.[3] Cucurbita seed oil contains a number of these, including about 25% oleic acid and 55% linoleic acid.[5]

No satisfactory clinical evidence presently attests to the utility of either cucurbita seed or seed oil in treating prostatic enlargement. As a matter of fact, there is no more evidence to support such claims than for other deceptive claims made about the efficacy of a mixture of amino acids (glycine, alanine, and glutamic acid) in relieving the same condition. Surgical intervention is usually necessary if the degree of benign (nonmalignant) prostatic enlargement is enough to cause appreciable urinary retention.[6]

Cucurbita seeds are an effective teniafuge, but strain differences in cucurbitin content make it very difficult to know how much should be taken to get results. Although toxicity or undesirable side effects associated with cucurbita seeds have not been reported in the literature, it is not easy, since it varies so, to recommend the unstandardized drug for treatment of intestinal worms. It is impossible to recommend it for prostate problems.

REFERENCES

1. V. E. Tyler, L. R. Brady, and J. E. Robbers: Pharmacognosy, 8th Ed. Lea & Febiger, Philadelphia, 1981, p. 479.
2. H. W. Felter and J. U. Lloyd: King's American Dispensatory, 18th Ed., Vol. 2. The Ohio Valley Co., Cincinnati, 1900, pp. 1443–1444.
3. K. W. Donsbach: Your Prostate, International Institute of Natural Health Sciences, Huntington Beach, Calif., 1976, pp. 2–4.
4. V. H. Mihranian and C. I. Abou-Chaar: Lloydia 31: 23–29, 1968.
5. H. A. Hoppe: Drogenkunde, 8th Ed., Vol. 1. Walter de Gruyter, Berlin, 1975, pp. 368–369.
6. G. S. Avery, Ed.: Drug Treatment, 2nd Ed. Adis Press, Sydney, Australia, 1980, p. 825.

DAMIANA

Damiana, from the leaves of the Mexican shrub *Turnera diffusa* Willd. var. *aphrodisiaca* Urb., family Turneraceae, was introduced into American medicine in the fall of 1874 by a Washington, D.C. druggist who sold 8-oz. bottles of the tincture for $2 each.[1] The product was touted as a powerful aphrodisiac "to improve the sexual ability of the enfeebled and aged." It was said to have a specific effect on all the organs of the pelvis and to give "increased tone and activity to all the secretions in that vicinity." Stories of Mexican men who had sired children at very advanced ages were circulated to substantiate these claims.[2]

Within very few months, the reported activities of the drug were recognized as fraudulent,[3] but more than a century has scarcely diminished damiana's reputation in the minds of people who want to believe in its tonic and stimulating properties. Any physiological activity in various proprietary damiana preparations marketed around the turn of the century (e.g., Nyal's Compound Extract of Damiana) was actually due to the presence of other drugs, such as coca or nux vomica, and to a high alcoholic content, usually about 50%.[4]

Modern popular writers on drugs indicate that damiana leaves, drunk in the form of a tea or smoked like tobacco, produced a relaxed state in the user and a kind of subtle high with sexual overtones, somewhat reminiscent of the effects of marihuana.[5] The drug is supposed to be especially effective in women. Damiana liqueurs, produced in Mexico and subtly advertised as aphrodisiacs, contain only minute quantities of the drug. The amount is sufficient, however, to give these beverages a distinctive flavor.

Chemical studies have shown that damiana contains between 0.2 and 0.9% of a complex volatile oil which is responsible for most of the characteristic odor and taste of the drug. In addition, quantities of a resin, a bitter principle, tannin, mucilage, starch, etc. are present.[6] The reported presence of caffeine requires verifying. No constituent responsible for claims of damiana as an aphrodisiac has ever been identified. On the basis of available evidence, we must conclude that the drug lacks significant physiological activity and that no basis exists for its consumption by human beings. Indeed, the purported virtue of the product has been described as nothing more than an "herbal hoax."[7]

REFERENCES

1. Anon.: American Journal of Pharmacy 47: 426–427, 1875.
2. J. M. Maisch: Ibid. 47: 380–381, 1875.
3. *Idem.: Ibid.* 47: 429–430, 1875.
4. Nostrums and Quackery, 2nd Ed., Vol. 1. American Medical Association, Chicago, 1912, p. 537.
5. High Times Encyclopedia of Recreational Drugs. Stonehill Publishing Co., New York, 1978, pp. 106–107.
6. H. A. Hoppe: Drogenkunde, 8th Ed., Vol. 1. Walter de Gruyter, Berlin, 1975, p. 1096.
7. V. E. Tyler: Pharmacy in History 25: 55–60, 1983.

DANDELION

It is useful in treating warts, fungus infections, external and internal malignant growths, ulceration of the urinary passages, and obstructions of the liver, gallbladder, and spleen. It's a laxative, a stomach remedy, a promoter of healthy circulation, a skin toner, and a blood vessel cleanser and strengthener. It cures rheumatism, badly affected arthritic joints, and it's a marvelous tonic. It makes a fine wine, a great beer, an excellent coffee substitute, as well as a good food for birds, bees, pigs, rabbits, and people.[1] What is it? The newest miracle drug or manna from heaven? No! It's the common dandelion. After reading this description of that plant's virtues by herbal advocate William Smith, I even felt guilty about mowing my lawn.

Dandelion is one plant which probably requires no description. Its basal rosette of toothy leaves which rises from a hollow scape or flower stem capped by a deep yellow head of ligulate flowers makes *Taraxacum officinale* Wiggers (family Compositae) one of our best known weeds. A native of Europe, it is ubiquitous in North America. What is not generally known is that there are literally hundreds of forms or subspecies of the plant which vary sufficiently in appearance from each other to be recognized by botanical specialists.[2]

A large number of constituents have been isolated from the underground parts (rhizome and roots) of dandelion, but it is difficult to attribute much therapeutic utility to any of them. An undefined bitter principle, designated taraxacin, apparently has some favorable influence on the digestive process, but the compound responsible for the mild laxative action of the drug is unknown.[3] In small animal experiments, extracts of the leaves have exhibited a pronounced diuretic action, but again, the responsible principle(s) remains unidentified.[4] A proprietary product consisting of the expressed milky latex of dandelion herb is marketed in Germany where it is recommended for liver ailments,[5] but evidence for its effectiveness here is scanty.

In summary, no significant therapeutic benefits should be expected from the use of any dandelion products. The roots may stimulate the appetite a bit and aid digestion, as well as produce a slight laxative effect. Leaves of the plant may also have a transient diuretic action. However, many persons do enjoy dandelion greens, and they are a fairly good source of vitamin A. My personal experience with dandelion wine enhanced my appreciation of the California jug varieties without dandelions. Some say that the roasted root provides a tasty coffee substitute. These culinary applications far outweigh any medicinal uses for this common plant. I guess it's all right to mow my weedy lawn after all.

REFERENCES

1. W. Smith: Wonders in Weeds. Health Science Press, Bradford, England, 1977, pp. 66–68.
2. L. H. Bailey and E. Z. Bailey: Hortus Third. Macmillan, New York, 1976, p. 1097.
3. P. H. List and L. Hörhammer, Eds.: Hagers Handbuch der Pharmazeutischen Praxis, 4th Ed., Vol. 6C. Springer-Verlag, Berlin, 1979, pp. 16–21.
4. E. Rácz-Kotilla, G. Rácz, and A. Solomon: Planta Medica 26: 212–217, 1974.
5. Rote Liste 1981, Editio Cantor KG, Aulendorf/Württ., 1981, index no. 28 005.

DEVIL'S CLAW

"What's this devil's claw good for?
"Rheumatism. It's really good!"
"I never heard of it. If it's so good why don't
they sell it in drugstores?"
"They can't. The FDA won't approve it. If
they did, it would put all the doctors out of
business."

Conversation in an Orlando,
Florida, "health food" store.

D evil's claw consists of the secondary storage roots of *Harpagophytum procumbens* DC., a South African plant belonging to the family Pedaliaceae. The common name is derived from the plant's peculiar fruits which seem to be covered with miniature grappling hooks. Devil's claw, the name commonly used in the United States, is actually a translation of the German Teufelskralle; English synonyms include wood spider and grapple plant.[1]

The drug has been recommended for treating a wide variety of conditions including diseases of the liver, kidneys, and bladder, as well as allergies, arteriosclerosis, lumbago, gastrointestinal disturbances, menstrual difficulties, neuralgia, headache, climacteric (change of life) problems, heartburn, nicotine poisoning, and above all, rheumatism and arthritis.[2] The allegation that devil's claw induces abortion[3] remains unverified. It may be based on a misinterpretation of a statement by Watt and Breyer-Brandwijk that the drug is used by African natives to alleviate pain in pregnant women and especially in those anticipating a difficult delivery.[4] Even discounting this property, enough therapeutic activities have been attributed to devil's claw to cause some to consider it a "wonder" drug.

A limited clinical study carried out in Germany reported, in 1976, that devil's claw exhibited anti-inflammatory activity comparable in many respects to the well-known anti-arthritic drug, phenylbutazone. Analgesic effects were also observed along with reductions in abnormally high cholesterol and uric-acid blood levels.[2] Unfortunately, this is apparently the only study in animals or humans to demonstrate positive anti-inflammatory activity. Several investigators have tested the efficacy of devil's claw in various standard inflammation models in animals. Little or no activity was observed by any of them. Another clinical trial in arthritic patients showed no significant improvement after six weeks of treatment.[5]

Whatever anti-inflammatory effects devil's claw may possess are usually attributed to an iridoid glycoside designated harpagoside which is contained in commercial extracts of the root in concentrations of about 2%. This compound has been shown to be relatively nontoxic in small animal tests of short duration. Thus, as far as is now known, devil's claw appears to be a relatively safe herb, but there is very little scientific or clinical evidence to support its use in the treatment of rheumatism, arthritis, or any such inflammatory condition.

REFERENCES

1. O. H. Volk: Deutsche Apotheker-Zeitung 104: 573–576, 1964.
2. R. Kämpf: Schweizerische Apotheker-Zeitung 114: 337–342, 1976.
3. M. Abramowicz, Ed.: Medical Letter on Drugs and Therapeutics 21(7): 30, 1979.
4. J. M. Watt and M. G. Breyer-Brandwijk: The Medicinal and Poisonous Plants of Southern and Eastern Africa, 2nd Ed. E. & S. Livingstone Ltd., Edinburgh, 1962, p. 830.
5. Anon.: Lawrence Review 5: 5–6, 1984.

DONG QUAI

Dong quai or tang kuei consists of the root of the Chinese plant *Angelica polymorpha* Maxim. var *sinensis* Oliv., a member of the family Umbelliferae. The drug is mildly laxative, although it is used primarily for its uterine tonic, anti-spasmodic, and alternative (blood purifying) effects.[1]

It is recommended by modern herbalists for the treatment of almost every gynecological ailment, including menstrual cramps, irregularity or retarded flow, and weakness during the menstrual period. Dong quai is also said to bring relief from the symptoms of menopause but should not be used during pregnancy. In addition, it is thought to be a useful antispasmodic and of value in the treatment of hypertension. Its reputation also extends to blood "purification" and nourishment," and finally, to treating constipation.[2]

Under chemical investigation, seven different coumarin derivatives have been identified in dong quai, including oxypeucedanin, osthol, imperatorin, psoralen, and bergapten.[3] Many coumarins are known to act as vasodilators and antispasmodics; others, such as osthol, have a stimulating action on the central nervous system.[4] Thus at least some of the purported activities of dong quai can be accounted for by these compounds.

However, large doses of coumarins are not without undesirable effects, and the furocoumarins, such as psoralen and bergapten, are prone to cause photosensitization which may result in a type of dermatitis in persons exposed to them. Recently, some investigators have concluded that these so-called psoralens present sufficient risks to humans that all unnecessary exposure to them should be avoided.[5] For this reason, large amounts of a coumarin-containing drug such as dong quai cannot be recommended. Since every condition for which it is advocated is amenable to therapy with drugs known to be both safe and effective, there is really no reason to take dong quai as a medicinal agent.

REFERENCES

1. A. Barefoot Doctor's Manual. Running Press, Philadelphia, 1977, p. 721.

2. M. Tierra: The Way of Herbs. Unity Press, Santa Cruz, Calif., 1980. pp. 124–125.
3. K. Hata, M. Kozawa, and Y. Ikeshiro: Yakugaku Zasshi 87: 464–465, 1967.
4. E. Steinegger and R. Hänsel: Lehrbuch der Pharmakognosie, 3rd Ed. Springer-Verlag, Berlin, 1972, pp. 132–135.
5. G. W. Ivie, D. L. Holt, and M. C. Ivey: Science 213: 909–910, 1981.

ECHINACEA

Thoughtful readers may often wonder how mankind discovered the medicinal virtues of so many different plants. After teaching about drugs from natural sources for several years at the University of Nebraska, I knew the answer. Every few weeks during the summer months, another package would arrive in the mail containing some fragments of the woody rhizome and roots of a "peculiar" plant which, as explained in the accompanying letter, caused an unusual, acrid, tingling sensation on the tongue when it was chewed. Some Nebraska farmer, like most of his breed a close observer of nature, had once again discovered a potentially useful plant by the age-old process of trial and error.

I responded to all such inquiries with a much-used form letter identifying the plant source as *Echinacea angustifolia* DC., usually referred to simply as echinacea, or cone flower, or purple cone flower. This perennial member of the daisy family (Compositae), with its narrow leaves and stout stem up to 3 feet in height, terminating in a single, large purplish flower head, is native to the central United States. A similar species, *E. purpurea* (L.) Moench, distinguished by its somewhat broader leaves but apparently possessing similar properties, is also used as a drug.

Appropriately enough, echinacea was first introduced into medicine by a Nebraskan, Dr. H. C. F. Meyer of Pawnee City. Having learned of the therapeutic value of the drug from the Indians about 1871, Meyer used it to prepare a "blood purifier" which he claimed was useful in treating almost any condition including rheumatism, migraine, erysipelas (streptococcus infections), dyspepsia, pain, wounds, sores, eczema, dizziness, sore eyes, poisoning by herbs, rattlesnake bites, tumors, syphilis, gangrene, typhoid, malaria, diphtheria, bee stings, hydrophobia, and hemorrhoids.[1] In 1885, Meyer called the attention of a pharmaceutical manufacturer, Lloyd Brothers of Cincinnati, to the drug, and that firm subsequently introduced several echinacea products intended primarily as anti-infective agents. By 1920, echinacea was the firm's most popular plant drug, but with the advent of the sulfa drugs in the 1930's, it began to fall into disuse. No longer valued in conventional medicine, the drug continues to be employed in folk medicine, either taken internally to increase the body's resistance to various types of infections or applied locally for its wound-healing action.[2]

Echinacea contains about 0.1% of a caffeic acid glycoside designated echinacoside which does possess definite bacteriostatic properties.[3] The pungent principle in the drug was found to be a complex isobutylamide and designated echinacein. Interestingly enough, it possesses significant insecticidal activity, especially against houseflies.[4] More recently, a hydrocarbon isolated from echinacea root and identified as (Z)-1,8-pentadecadiene has been shown to possess antitumor activity.[5]

Evidence continues to accumulate to support the use of this drug as an anti-infective and wound-healing agent. Echinacea's immunostimulant effects are now attributed to at least two high molecular weight polysaccharides, a heteroxylan and an arabin-orhamnogalactan.[6] These, and possibly other similar constituents, apparently act by three different mechanisms: stimulating phagocytosis, increasing respiratory activity, and causing increased mobility of the leucocytes. This may result in both a subjective and objective normalization of the body's general condition and a clear improvement in such conditions as the common cold, sore throat, and general debilitation.[7]

Much more work on the constituents and potential hazards of echinacea is required before a definite statement can be made regarding its utility as a modern therapeutic agent. However, it is a plant drug that is certainly worthy of continued attention by scientists and clinicians.

Persons wishing to obtain quantities of echinacea should be aware that a very high percentage of the root currently marketed is not either *Echinacea angustifolia* or *E. purpurea* but is instead obtained from another member of the composite family, *Parthenium integrifolium* L. Such widespread adulteration with a cheaper, inactive substitute, actually threatens the integrity of echinacea as a medicinal plant.[8]

REFERENCES

1. J. U. Lloyd: A Treatise on Echinacea. Lloyd Brothers, Cincinnati, 1924.
2. M. Grieve: A Modern Herbal, Vol. 1. Dover Publications, New York, 1971, p. 265.
3. P. H. List and L. Hörhammer, Eds.: Hagers Handbuch der Pharmazeutischen Praxis, 4th Ed., Vol. 4, Springer-Verlag, Berlin, 1973, pp. 751–754.
4. M. Jacobson: Journal of Organic Chemistry 32: 1646–1647, 1967.

5. D. J. Voaden and M. Jacobson: Journal of Medicinal Chemistry 15: 619–623, 1972.
6. H. Wagner: *In* Natural Products and Drug Development, P. Krogs-gaard-Larsen, S. B. Christensen and H. Kofod, Eds. Munksgaard, Copenhagen, 1984, pp. 391–404.
7. G. Harnischfeger: Deutsche Apotheker Zeitung 125: 1295–1296, 1985.
8. S. Foster: Echinacea Exalted!, 2nd Ed., Ozark Beneficial Plant Project, Brixley, Missouri, 1985, p. 11.

EVENING PRIMROSE

Native to North America, where it is regarded as a noxious weed, the evening primrose (*Oenothera biennis L.*) is considered by some authorities to be a complex of several closely related species. This biennial herb, a member of the family Onagraceae, produces a large number of highly fertile seeds which are responsible for its introduction and establishment in Europe from ships' ballast in the first years of the seventeenth century. Although the native Indians and early European settlers in America used the whole plant for a variety of conditions ranging from asthmatic coughs to gastrointestinal disorders to bruises, it is the fatty oil obtained from the small, reddish brown seeds that has caused a resurgence of interest in this herb.[1]

Evening primrose seeds yield about 14% of fixed oil which, in turn, contains approximately 9% of an unusual constituent, *cis*-gamma-linolenic acid (GLA). GLA is a known precursor of prostaglandin E_1, serving as a key intermediate in the biosynthetic pathway leading from *cis*-linolenic acid to that prostaglandin. In fact, conversion of the predominant, essential dietary fatty acid, linolenic acid, to GLA is apparently a limiting step in prostaglandin production. Advocates of the use of evening primrose oil claim that increased intake of it produces a large number of beneficial effects including, but not limited to, weight loss without dieting, lowered blood cholesterol, lowered blood pressure, cure of rheumatoid arthritis, relief of premenstrual pain, slowed progression of multiple sclerosis, and even the alleviation of hangovers.[2]

Such claims require extensive clinical testing before they can be verified. Scientifically, they would be valid only if all of the specified conditions are favorably influenced by additional production in the body of prostaglandin E_1 and if a deficiency of PGA is the single factor responsible for limited prostaglandin production. Both of these factors remain unproven. If they are not true, then assumptions of the efficacy of evening primrose oil in such conditions is somewhat like assuming one's car will run better if the gas tank is completely full instead of only half full.

The extravagant claims made by proponents of the use of evening primrose oil as a veritable cure-all should, nevertheless, not obscure the fact that it has been shown in several clinical studies to hold some promise as a useful therapeutic agent. For example, a double-blind, controlled cross-over study of the effect of oral doses of the oil in 99 patients with atopic (allergic) eczema showed that the product produced significant clinical improvement when taken in high doses (6 grams per day in adults) over a 12-week period.[3] In an uncontrolled study involving treatment of 291 patients with mastalgia (painful breasts), 45% of those receiving 3 grams per day of evening primrose oil for 3 to 6 months obtained excellent results, but 21% of the responders relapsed after one course of treatment. Still, such positive results are encouraging and should prompt additional studies.

Evening primrose oil is expensive, presently retailing at about 1 cent per milligram of contained GLA. Consumers should be aware that some of the products on the market may be adulterated with cheaper oils (soy or safflower), or they may be biologically useless due to decomposition.[5] The finding that seeds of the European black current, *Ribes nigrum* L., contain about 6% GLA, in comparison to less than 2% in evening primrose seeds, has now resulted in the appearance on the market of products containing the fixed oil of this plant.[6] If GLA should eventually prove to be a useful therapeutic agent, better sources than evening primrose seed will certainly be required.

REFERENCES

1. C. J. Briggs: Canadian Pharmaceutical Journal 119: 248–254, 1986.
2. R. A. Passwater: Evening Primrose Oil, Kent Publishing, Inc., New Canaan, Conn., 1981, 30 pp.
3. S. Wright and J. L. Burton: Lancet II: 1120–1122, 1982.
4. J. K. Pye, R. E. Mansel, and L. E. Hughes: Lancet II: 373–377, 1985.
5. Anon.: Lawrence Review of Natural Products 5(3): 11, 1984.
6. H. Traitler, H. Winter, U. Richli, and Y. Ingenbleek: Lipids 19: 923–928, 1984.

EYEBRIGHT

Any discussion of this herb must begin with the problems surrounding its name which are both numerous and difficult. The common name, eyebright, refers to species of *Euphorbia*, *Lobelia*, and *Sabbatia*, as well as to the plant considered here, *Euphrasia officinalis* L. (family Scrophulariaceae). However, many botanists, particularly those of Continental Europe, believe that *E. officinalis* L. represents some four different species and that the plants used medically include *E. rostkoviana* Hayne, *E. stricta* Host, and others. As far as we know, these closely related plants, which do vary slightly in their botanical features, are nevertheless quite similar chemically. It would therefore seem useful, if not entirely accurate, to continue to designate them by the older, more inclusive title, *E. officinalis* L.

Eyebright is a small, annual plant with deeply cut leaves, native to the heaths and pastures of Britain and Europe; from July to September it displays many small, white or purplish flowers variegated with yellow. The various spots and stripes on the flowers cause them to resemble bloodshot, or similarly afflicted, eyes. This, in turn, has caused the plant to be used since the Middle Ages to treat such conditions.[1] The usage was obviously based on the so-called Doctrine of Signatures.

In his epic poem, *Paradise Lost*, Milton describes how the Archangel Michael used "euphrasy" (eyebright) to clear Adam's sight after his visual nerve had been clouded as a result of eating the "false fruit." This testifies to the popularity of the drug during the latter half of the 17th century when Milton was writing his most famous work.

Most modern herbalists recommend a lotion or infusion, prepared from the entire overground portion of the plant for conjunctivitis and other eye irritations.[2-4] The ancient writers, such as Culpeper and Parkinson, also advised internal consumption of the herb for treatment of similar conditions.[5]

Chemical studies of eyebright have identified a number of constituents including aucubin, caffeic and ferulic acids, sterols, choline, various basic compounds, and a volatile oil.[6] But none of these constituents is known to possess any useful therapeutic properties for the treatment of eye disease, nor are there any modern scientific studies which attempt to measure the effectiveness of the drug. Furthermore, the instillation or application of any nonsterile solution to the eye involves considerable risk of potential infection and should never be advocated or condoned. The practice is particularly hazardous if the nonsterile, home-made lotion contains a large number of principles of unknown safety or efficacy. For this reason, ophthalmic application of eye-bright, as advocated by modern herbalists, is definitely not recommended.

REFERENCES

1. M. Grieve: A Modern Herbal, Vol. 1. Dover Publications, New York, 1971, pp. 290–293.
2. F. and V. Mitton: Mitton's Practical Herbal. W. Foulsham & Co., Ltd., London, 1976, p. 86.
3. W. H. Hylton, Ed.: The Rodale Herb Book, Rodale Press Book Div., Emmaus, Pa., 1974, pp. 437–438.
4. M. Stuart, Ed.: The Encyclopedia of Herbs and Herbalism, Grosset & Dunlap, New York, 1979, p. 189.
5. R. C. Wren and R. W. Wren: Potter's New Cyclopaedia of Botanical Drugs and Preparations, New Ed. Health Science Press, Hengiscote, England, 1975, pp. 118–19.
6. K. J. Harkiss and P. Timmins: Planta Medica 23: 342–347, 1973.

FENNEL

Because of its pleasant, aromatic odor and its reputation as a stomachic or aid to digestion, fennel is a well-known and widely used folk remedy. The plant, *Foeniculum vulgare* Mill., is a tall (up to 5 ft.), perennial herb with feathery, almost thread-like, leaves and yellow flowers; it is a member of the family Umbelliferae. There are numerous cultivated varieties. The dried ripe fruits are the part used for their medicinal virtues, but since they are rather small, they are often referred to as seeds.[1]

Fennel has been recommended for the treatment of a variety of ailments but chiefly as a carminative, that is, an agent which helps expel gas to relieve flatulence. It has often been combined with various purgatives (see senna, for example) to reduce their tendency to cause griping.[2] The drug has a reputation for loosening phlegm and is a common ingredient in cough preparations in Europe. Fennel water is commonly given to infants there to relieve colic and also for its reputed calmative effects.[3]

A large number of constituents have been identified in fennel, but its desirable stomachic and carminative properties are attributed primarily to the volatile oil which exists in the fruits to the extent of about 2 to 6%. This oil consists mostly (50 to 90%) of *trans*-anethole with smaller amounts of fenchone (up to 20%), estragole, limonene, camphene, and α-pinene. Producing essentially the same actions as the fruit, the oil has been shown to exert spasmolytic (relieves spasms) effects on smooth muscles of experimental animals.[4] This may partially explain fennel's effectiveness as a carminative.

Both fennel fruit and particularly fennel oil are widely employed as fragrance components in a variety of cosmetic preparations and as flavors in foods, beverages, condiments, and the like. There is little question of their safety when used in the very small amounts required for such purposes. Fennel fruit itself, in quantities normally utilized for medicinal teas or similar preparations, is innocuous except for producing a rare allergic response. Fennel volatile oil is quite a different matter. Quantities as small as 1 to 5 ml. have caused not only skin irritation but vomiting, seizures, and respiratory problems such as pulmonary edema.[5] For this reason, self-medication with fennel should be restricted to appropriate use of the fruits (seeds); the volatile oil should not be used.

REFERENCES

1. H. W. Youngken: Textbook of Pharmacognosy, 6th Ed. The Blakiston Co., Philadelphia, 1948, pp. 614–617.
2. M. Grieve: A Modern Herbal, Vol. 1. Dover Publications, New York, 1971, pp. 293–297.
3. M. Pahlow: Das grosse Buch der Heilpflanzen. Gräfe und Unzer GmbH, Munich, 1979, pp. 135–136.
4. A. Y. Leung: Encyclopedia of Common Natural Ingredients Used in Food, Drugs, and Cosmetics. John Wiley & Sons, New York, 1980, pp. 169–170.
5. D. G. Spoerke, Jr.: Herbal Medications, Woodbridge Press, Santa Barbara, Calif., 1980, p. 70.

FENUGREEK

Fenugreek consists of the dried ripe seeds of a small, southern European herb known technically as *Trigonella foenum-graecum* L., a member of the family Leguminosae. It is variously referred to as trigonella or as Greek hay seed. The seeds contain up to 40% of a mucilage causing them to be used in various poultices and ointments intended for external application. Fenugreek has also been administered internally for stomach ailments, again due to its soothing mucilaginous properties. The taste of the seed, somewhat reminiscent of maple sugar, accounts for its use as a spice and a flavoring agent, especially in imitation maple syrup.[1] Fenugreek is soothing, flavorful, and even nutritious. Although it is not a particularly potent medicament, it is quite harmless in normal use.

Lydia Pinkham's Vegetable Compound, according to the original formula in her own handwriting, contained fenugreek as its principal ingredient — other than alcohol. Twelve ounces of the seed were combined with 8 ounces of unicorn root (*Aletris farinosa* L.) and 6 ounces each of life root (*Senecio aureus* L.), black cohosh [*Cimicifuga racemosa* (L.) Nutt.] and pleurisy root (*Asclepias tuberosa* L.) in enough alcohol to make 100 pints of this old-time panacea.[2] Neither fenugreek nor any of the other ingredients is sufficiently active to account for the remarkable properties attributed to the Vegetable Compound in some of the verses still sung by college students and other irreverent types:

> "Widow Brown she had no children,
> Though she loved them very dear;
> So she took some Vegetable Compound,
> Now she has them twice a year."

> *Chorus*

> "Let us sing of Lydia Pinkham,
> And her love for the human race;
> How she sells her Vegetable Compound
> And the papers publish her face."

REFERENCES

1. F. Rosengarten, Jr.: The Book of Spices, Rev. Ed. Pyramid Books, New York, 1973, pp. 238–243.
2. S. Stage: Female Complaints, W. W. Norton, New York, 1979, p. 89.

FEVERFEW

Since the time of Dioscorides (78 A.D.) feverfew has been used for the treatment of headache, menstrual irregularities, stomachache, and especially, fevers. In fact, its common name is simply a corruption of the Latin *febrifugia* or fever reducer. The proper scientific name of this strongly aromatic, perennial herb, of the family Compositae is a matter of disagreement among botanists. At different times it has been placed in five different genera! Presently, *Chrysanthemum parthenium* (L.) Bernh. seems to be the designation most widely accepted in the United States.

In the 1970's, persons unable to obtain relief from the painful symptoms of migraine and arthritis by conventional means began to turn to feverfew as an alternative therapy. Consumption of only 2 or 3 fresh leaves daily for prolonged periods was found, for example, to decrease the frequency as well as the pain of migraine attacks. Considerable evidence has now been obtained from studies with fresh whole leaves, freezedried powdered leaves, and leaf extracts to confirm feverfew's effectiveness in such cases.[2,3] However, neither the identity of the plant's active principle(s) nor its mechanism of action has been established with certainty.

Several theories explaining its mechanism of action have been proposed, but recent studies on feverfew as a prophylactic treatment for migraine postulate that the observed effects may be attributed to the plant's content of sesquiterpene lactones.[4] Some compounds of this type are known to be spasmolytic. That is, they render the smooth muscles in the walls of the cerebral blood vessels less reactive to certain compounds that normally occur in the body and have a pronounced influence on them. Such so-called endogenous substances include norepinephrine, prostaglandins, and serotonin. Thus the active compound(s) might produce its antimigraine effect in a manner similar to methysergide (Sansert®), a known serotonin antagonist.

Regardless of its mode of action, feverfew appears to be a potentially valuable herbal remedy for the treatment of migraine and, possibly, arthritis as well. However, some caution must be observed with respect to the purchase and use of certain commercially available feverfew tablets, some of which have been found to contain only a small percentage of the labeled amount of active plant material.[5] Long-term toxicity tests are urgently needed to establish the herb's safety. It would also be highly desirable to identify the active constituent(s) in feverfew as well as to carry out additional clinical tests aimed at discovering the range of modern uses of this ancient herb.[6]

REFERENCES

1. M. I. Berry: Pharmaceutical Journal 232: 611–614, 1984.
2. A. N. Makheja and J. M. Bailey: Lancet II: 1054, 1981.
3. S. Heptinstall, L. Williamson, A. White, and J. R. A. Mitchell: Lancet I: 1071–1074, 1985.
4. E. S. Johnson, N. P. Kadam. D. M. Hylands, and P. J. Hylands: British Medical Journal 291: 569–573, 1985.
5. W. A. Groenewegen and S. Heptinstall: Lancet I: 44–45, 1986.
6. V. E. Tyler: Pharmacy International 7: 205, 1986.

FO-TI (HO SHOU-WU)

"What's in a name? that which we call a rose
By any other name would smell as sweet;"
William Shakespeare
Romeo and Juliet
Act II, Scene II

Most of the recent herb catalogs list a botanical called fo-ti, sometimes with a cross-reference to ho shou-wu which many authors insist is the proper title for this drug. Both names refer to the dried tuberous root of *Polygonum multiflorum* Thunb., an evergreen climbing plant of the family Polygonaceae, native to Japan and widely used as a folk remedy in Chinese medicine.

The reason some writers[1] object to the designation fo-ti for this plant is its potential confusion with the herbal mixture marketed as Fo-ti Tieng®. That product, which has a registered trademark name, is totally different from fo-ti or ho shou-wu. Fo-ti Tieng® consists of a mixture of the leaves and stems of a diminutive variety of gotu kola [*Centella asiatica* (L.) Urb. of the family Umbelliferae], the root of meadowsweet [*Gillenia trifoliata* (L.) Moench of the family Rosaceae] which has both emetic and laxative properties, and small amounts of caffeine-containing cola or kolanuts, the dried cotyledons of *Cola nitida* (Vent.) Schott et Endl., family Sterculiaceae, or related species.[2] Since whatever activity the mixture may possess is probably due mostly to the gotu kola contained in it, the reader is referred to the section on that drug in this book for details.

If all of these nomenclatural similarities seem confusing, and they are, keep in mind that these drug names, and others as well, may have been created on purpose to confuse the consumer into paying a relatively high price for a cheaper but similarly named product. In any event, the one we are discussing here is most commonly called fo-ti, less commonly ho shou-wu, and is the root of *Polygonum multiflorum*.

The Chinese apparently believe that the root exhibits quite different properties according to its size and the age of the plant from which it is derived.[3] Essentially, the older the better: Use of 50-year-old root preserves one's natural hair color; 100-year-old root helps one maintain a cheerful appearance; 150-year-old root causes new teeth to grow; 200-year-old-root preserves one's youth and energy; and the 300-year-old product makes one immortal. Needless to say, very little (if any) of the truly ancient product is available.

A more realistic appraisal of the use of fo-ti was provided by the American Herbal Pharmacology Delegation in the 1975 report of its visit to the People's Republic of China.[4] That group noted the drug was used alone for scrofula (tuberculosis of the lymph glands), cancer, and constipation and mixed with other medicinals, for liver and spleen weakness, vertigo, and insomnia. There is an old report in the European literature mentioning the effectiveness of the drug in treating diabetes,[5] but it is interesting that it is apparently not employed for this purpose in China.

Chemical studies of fo-ti have revealed the presence of chrysophanol and emodin (both in the free state and combined as glycosides) together with a small amount of rhein.[6] All of these anthraquinone derivatives possess cathartic properties which account for the drug's noted effectiveness in the treatment of constipation. This is probably the only real action of fo-ti, at least as far as is presently known. However, other species of *Polygonum* do contain leucoanthocyanidins which possess anti-inflammatory activity, decrease blood coagulability, and have various cardiovascular effects.[4] It is possible that some of these compounds may eventually be discovered in fo-ti. Until then, the drug must be categorized simply as a laxative with various undetermined side effects.

REFERENCES

1. D. Mowrey: Herbalist 5(1): 14–15, 1980
2. V. E. Tyler, L. R. Brady, and J. E. Robbers: Pharmacognosy, 8th Ed. Lea & Febiger, Philadelphia, 1981, p. 482.
3. C. Lam: Herbalist 2(7): 13–14, 1977.
4. Herbal Pharmacology in the People's Republic of China. National Academy of Sciences, Washington, D.C., 1975, p. 186.
5. O. A. F. Gnadt: Die Pharmazie 1: 103–107, 1946.
6. P. H. List and L. Hörhammer, Eds.: Hagers Handbuch der Pharmazeutischen Praxis, 4th Ed. Vol. 6A. Springer-Verlag, Berlin, 1977, p. 823.

GARLIC AND OTHER ALLIUMS

Even relatively well-informed readers, asked to name the most popular herbal panacea or cure-all, might be inclined to say ginseng. They would be wrong. As broad as its claims of curative properties are, ginseng's hypothesized range of therapeutic and overall use, until recently limited primarily to the Orient, do not begin to compare with the many and varied worldwide applications of garlic and its near relatives, onions, leeks, and shallots. These well known members of the lily family (Liliaceae) all belong to the genus *Allium*; garlic is *A. sativum* L., onion is *A. cepa* L., the leek is *A. ampeloprasum* L., and the shallot is *A. ascalonicum* L.

The bulbs and occasionally the leaves of these plants, designated collectively as alliums, have been used by people since the earliest days of recorded history as both food and medicine. Keller[1] has listed some 125 different uses of the alliums, only one of which is for culinary purposes. Some of the others are very broad categories indeed, such as, cures "all diseases." Others are contradictory—cures "hypertension" and "low blood pressure." Still others are more mythical than medical; garlic, for example, was noted for its ability to ward off vampires, demons, witches, and similar imaginary beings. Above all, the alliums were valued as aphrodisiacs, agents which produce sexual desire and improved performance.

Most of the modern folkloric medicinal use of these plants has focused on garlic. Although some advocates still recommend its use for everything from cancer and tuberculosis to hemorrhoids and athlete's foot,[2-4] the most frequent use of garlic in recent times has been in treating atherosclerosis and high blood pressure. A prominent secondary application is to provide relief from various stomach and intestinal ailments.[5]

The chemistry of garlic has been extensively investigated. Its bulbs contain an odorless, sulfur-containing amino acid derivative known as alliin (S-allyl-L-cysteine sulfoxide). This parent substance has no antibacterial properties, but when the bulbs are ground, alliin comes into contact with the enzyme allinase which converts it to allicin (diallyldisulfide-S-oxide), a potent antibacterial agent. Unfortunately, allicin is extremely odoriferous; it's the carrier of the typical garlic odor. It is also unstable, so when garlic bulbs are subjected to steam distillation to obtain their volatile oil (0.1 to 0.36%), some of it breaks down to yield diallyldisulfide and related garlic-smelling compounds.[6] Still, the allicin with its antibacterial activity against numerous gram-positive and gram-negative pathogenic organisms may account for the alleged effectiveness of garlic in the folk treatment of infectious conditions.

Beneficial effects of garlic on digestive disturbances and on the cardiovascular system have been demonstrated in animals and to some extent in human beings. Experiments showed that garlic inhibited experimental hypercholesterolemia (high blood cholesterol) in rabbits and reduced high blood pressure in both dogs and people. Small doses increased the tonus of the smooth muscles of the intestines, thereby increasing peristalsis, but large doses inhibited such movements.[5] Controlled studies carried out on volunteers in India showed that individuals consuming more than 50 grams of garlic or 600 grams of onions per week had significantly lower serum-triglycerides, beta lipoproteins, phospholipids, and plasma-fibrinogen levels than persons who had never eaten garlic or onions. There were indications that even moderate consumption of these products (up to 10 grams of garlic or 200 grams of onions weekly) reduced the blood levels of phospholipids and plasma-fibrinogen. The investigators concluded that regular consumption of onion and garlic in the diet had a protective effect on some important factors which influence atherosclerosis.[7]

The ability of garlic to provide some protection against atherosclerosis, coronary thrombosis, and stroke is believed to be directly related to its ability to inhibit aggregation of the blood platelets. This property, initially attributed to allicin, is now known to be due to a newly identified compound designated ajoene, a self-condensation product of allicin.[8,9] As an antithrombotic (clot-preventing) agent, ajoene is at least as potent as aspirin, and its activity is enhanced by two breakdown products which accompany it in garlic and which are also mildly antithrombotic.

As for onions, further research may eventually reveal the presence in them of ajoene-like compounds. The reported occurrence in onions of prostaglandin A_1 is of interest.[10] PGA_1 has the ability to decrease blood pressure when injected intravenously into small animals and humans. However, it is not known if the compound is active when taken by mouth. Further, its initial isolation from onions has not been independently verified. It seems more logical now to attempt to explain the beneficial effects of onions on the cardiovascular system on the basis of the presence of ajoene-like compounds rather than on the presence of prostaglandins.

Further pharmacological and chemical studies are required before the real therapeutic value of garlic, onions, leeks, and their relatives can be determined with certainty. In the meantime, we must conclude that their potential is considerable.

In spite of this potential, a word of caution is in order. Although heating apparently has no appreciable effect on garlic's antibacterial properties,[5] even the most ardent advocates of the plant agree that all the various ways of drying garlic invariably destroy some of its effects.[2] Ajoene, for example, has never been detected in either dehydrated garlic powder or in any of the various commercial garlic capsules, oils, extracts, or related preparations so far examined. Also, many of the garlic preparations marketed in "health food" stores contain "garlic oil" of unspecified composition which has been rendered tasteless and odorless by an unspecified process. Now keep in mind that the active antibacterial part of garlic oil consists of the odoriferous constituents. Therefore, if one wishes to obtain the so-called benefits of the alliums, one must consume them either in the fresh state or in some other condition (for instance, after freeze-drying) which alters the plant material as little as possible. Following this advice may reduce the number of one's close associates in direct proportion to the quantity and frequency of alliums consumed.

Still, based on current knowledge, there does seem to be a grain of truth in the old Welsh rhyme:

> "Eat leeks in March and wild garlic in May,
> And all the year after physicians may play."

REFERENCES

1. M. S. Keller: Mysterious Herbs & Roots. Peace Press, Culver City, Calif., 1978, pp. 162–211.
2. T. Watanabe: Garlic Therapy. Japan Publications, Tokyo, 1974.
3. G. J. Binding: About Garlic. Thorsons Publishers Ltd., Wellingborough, England, 1970.
4. P. Airola: The Miracle of Garlic. Health Plus, Phoenix, Ariz., 1978.
5. W. Petkov: Deutsche Apotheker-Zeitung 106: 1861–1867, 1966.

6. E. Steinegger and R. Hänsel: Lehrbuch der Pharmakognosie, 3rd Ed. Springer-Verlag, Berlin, 1972, pp. 423–425.
7. G. S. Sainani, D. B. Desai, and K. N. More: Lancet 2: 575–576, 1976.
8. E. Block, S. Ahmad, M. K. Jain, R. W. Crecely, R. Apitz-Castro, and M. R. Cruz: Journal of the American Chemical Society 106: 8295–8296, 1984.
9. E. Block: Scientific American 252(3): 114–119, 1985.
10. K. A. Attrep, W. P. Bellman, Sr., M. Attrep, Jr., J. B. Lee, and W. E. Braselton, Jr.: Lipids 15: 292–297, 1980.

GENTIAN

Bitter substances taken before eating are supposed to improve both the appetite and the digestion by increasing the flow of gastric juice. Although there is little evidence to support this view in normal, healthy persons, it is probably factual for those suffering from conditions such as anemia.[1] Nevertheless, many well people genuinely believe in the beneficial effects of so-called bitter stomachics.

The use of such old-time proprietary remedies as Hostetter's Celebrated Stomach Bitters in the United States has largely given way to adding a few drops of Angostura Bitters (which contains gentian, not angostura) to the evening cocktail. In Europe, various alcoholic beverages flavored with gentian and other bitter principles remain extremely popular and are widely consumed, especially before eating a heavy, fatty meal which may cause digestive difficulties. My friends in Germany recommend it and use it themselves before attacking a large, spit-roasted *Schweinshaxen* (pork shank) at a specialty restaurant like the Haxnbauer in Munich.

Gentian, the dried rhizome and roots (underground parts) of *Gentiana lutea* L. of the family Gentianaceae, a moderately tall, perennial herb with an erect stem and large, ovate leaves, is by far the most popular of the bitter stomachics. The plant has large flowers which grow in characteristic orange-yellow clusters. It is a native of the alpine and subalpine pastures of central and southern Europe and is extensively cultivated there.[2] The bitter alcoholic beverage prepared from it has become almost a trademark of specific regions in several European countries.

Modern herbalists extol the virtues of gentian far beyond those of a simple bitter. It is believed to be useful in the treatment of exhaustion from chronic disease and in cases of general debility as well. They view it as a strengthener of the human system — in other words, as a tonic. It is also said to be useful as a febrifuge (reduces fever), emmenagogue (stimulates the menstrual flow), anthelmintic (expels intestinal worms), and antiseptic. In their view, it is helpful in treating hysteria and in combination with other drugs, malaria.[3] Gentian is usually consumed in the form of a tea or as one of the commercially available alcoholic extracts.

Glycosides known as amarogentin and gentiopicrin are primarily responsible for the bitter taste of gentian. In addition, the plant contains several alkaloids (mainly gentianine and gentialutine), xanthones, triterpenes, and sugars. Aside from its action as a bitter stomachic, none of the other purported effects is well-documented in human beings. Some experiments on small animals indicate that gentian may increase the secretion of bile; the alkaloid gentianine also exhibits anti-inflammatory properties.[4]

Widespread use of gentian as an appetite stimulant and digestive aid would seem to favor the drug as effective for these conditions. However, since it is normally consumed as an alcoholic beverage, it is difficult to separate the effects of gentian from those of alcohol which are very similar, at least when the alcohol is consumed in moderate amounts.[5] In normal individuals, gentian is unlikely to produce undesirable side effects, but Pahlow warns that the drug may not be tolerated well by those with very high blood pressure or by expectant mothers.[6] Actually, these people should be very cautious about using any medication, herbal or otherwise.

REFERENCES

1. T. Sollmann: A Manual of Pharmacology, 7th Ed. W. B. Saunders, Philadelphia, 1948, pp. 167–168.
2. H. W. Youngken: Textbook of Pharmacognosy, 6th Ed. The Blakiston Co., Philadelphia, 1948, pp. 670–674.
3. M. Grieve: A Modern Herbal, Vol. 1. Dover Publications, New York, 1971, pp. 347–349.
4. A. Y. Leung: Encyclopedia of Common Natural Ingredients Used in Food, Drugs, and Cosmetics. John Wiley, New York, 1980, pp. 180–182.
5. T. Sollman: Op. cit., pp. 615–616.
6. M. Pahlow: Das grosse Buch der Heilpflanzen. Gräfe und Unzer GmbH, Munich, 1979, pp. 124–126.

GINGER

Ginger is technically a rhizome (underground stem) of the plant *Zingiber officinale* Roscoe of the family Zingiberaceae. In commerce it is frequently referred to as Jamaica ginger, African ginger, or Cochin ginger, according to its geographical origin. Ginger was known in China nearly 2500 years ago, and it continues to be valued throughout the world as a spice or flavoring agent.[1] However, it also has the reputation, particularly in Asian medicine, as a carminative (digestive aid), stimulant, diuretic, and antiemetic.

The characteristic aroma of ginger is due to a volatile oil which it contains in amounts of about 1 to 3%. Its pungency is attributed to ginger oleoresin (mixture of volatile oil and resin). Components of this oleoresin known as gingerols have recently been studied and found to possess cardiotonic, as well as antipyretic, analgesic, antitussive (anticough) and sedative properties when administered to laboratory animals.[2]

Comparatively little is known about the pharmacological effects of ginger in human beings. One double-blind study found that 940 mg. of powdered ginger was superior to the antihistamine dimenhydrinate (100 mg.) or a placebo in preventing nausea and vomiting in 36 subjects prone to motion sickness, who were tested while blindfolded in a rotating chair. In a 6-minute test, subjects who received doses of ginger remained in the chair an average of 5.5 minutes compared with 3.5 minutes for those receiving the antihistamine and 1.5 minutes for the placebo group. The authors postulate that unlike dimenhydrinate, which exerts its action on the central nervous system, ginger apparently acts by virtue of its aromatic, carminative, and absorbent properties directly on the gastrointestinal tract.[3] It would be highly desirable to attempt to verify the results of this single study by additional investigations.

Ginger-filled capsules have subsequently appeared on the market where they are advertised as providing protection against motion sickness. Pamphlets accompanying ginger tea also recommend its use for the same purpose. There are no reports of severe toxicity in humans from eating ginger, but some of the recent pharmacological studies of its constituents would seem to indicate that very large overdoses might carry the potential for causing depression of the central nervous system and cardiac arrhythmias. In the meantime, further investigations of the chemical constituents and the therapeutic properties of ginger are certainly warranted.

REFERENCES

1. V. E. Tyler, L. R. Brady, and J. E. Robbers: Pharmacognosy, 8th Ed. Lea & Febiger, Philadelphia, 1981, pp. 156–157.
2. Anon.: Lawrence Review of Natural Products, April, 1986.
3. D. B. Mowrey and D. E. Clayson: Lancet I: 655–657, 1982.

GINSENG AND RELATED DRUGS

That too much has been written about ginseng is a gross understatement. The Research Institute of the Office of [Ginseng] Monopoly, Republic of Korea, has cited and abstracted 1191 books and papers published on the drug between 1687 and 1975.[1] And since 1975, the volume of writing has increased enormously. To say that we now have a reasonable knowledge of the botany and chemistry of ginseng is a fact. Recent studies in both areas have made significant contributions to our knowledge. But to say that we have an adequate understanding of the way ginseng works (if indeed it does) in helping to maintain health or in preventing or curing disease in the human body is an enormous exaggeration. Most of the literature in this area is based more on superstition and subjective opinion than on objective, scientific evidence. *conclusion*

Nothing about ginseng seems to be totally free from controversy. Even the proper name of the low-growing, shade-loving perennial herbs of the family Araliaceae which yield the highly valued roots is not agreed upon by all specialists. Following American authorities,[2] we are using the designation *Panax pseudoginseng* Wallich to designate the species widely cultivated and utilized in the Orient. But remember, it is also known as *P. ginseng* C. A. Mey. and as *P. schinseng* Nees. The native American species which occurs more or less commonly in wooded areas from Quebec to Minnesota and south to Georgia and Oklahoma is known as *P. quinquefolius* L. It is so intensively sought in the United States that it has been declared an endangered species. Its collection and sale are subject to registration, permits, reports, a collector-education program, and an official ginseng season. The plant is also cultivated to some extent in this country, but it is a slow-growing and exacting crop requiring at least six years to produce a marketable root, so cultivation has not proven very popular.

Basically, ginseng has been used for centuries in the Orient, especially in China, Japan, Korea, and parts of the Soviet Union, as a cure-all or panacea. This usage no doubt stems from the "Doctrine of Signatures" because the root is often decidedly man-like in appearance and therefore useful in the treatment of all "man's afflictions." Farnsworth[3] has pointed out that the wildest use of the drug in those areas is not in curing a particular disease but in a supportive role to maintain health. In this regard, ginseng is analogous to the ubiquitous vitamin tablets here, but with one important addition. The drug is widely believed to have a favorable influence on sexual potency, in other words, to be an aphrodisiac. More recently, as ginseng consumption has galloped across the Western world, its adaptogenic effects are being emphasized. As an adaptogen, it is believed to produce a state of increased resistance of the body to stress, overcoming disease by building up our general vitality and strengthening our normal body functions.[4] Although such indirect effects are naturally somewhat difficult to verify scientifically, favorable modification by ginseng of the stress effects of temperature changes, diet, restraint, exercise, and the like have been recorded. Moreover, useful pharmacologic effects in such conditions as anemia, atherosclerosis, depression, diabetes, edema, hypertension, and ulcers have also been documented.[3] In one area, however, ginseng's purported beneficial effects remain unsubstantiated. There is no evidence of enhanced sexual experience or potency resulting from its use.[5]

The principles believed to be responsible for ginseng's activities are triterpenoid saponins which exist in the root in large numbers.[6] Again the nomenclature of these compounds is extremely confusing and complex, for some of the same ones were isolated by different groups of investigators and given different names. Then, too, there are differences in composition between the oriental and American ginseng species. The active saponins are called ginsenosides by Japanese and panaxosides by Russian scientists. Thus, we have at least 11 saponins in oriental ginseng, such as ginsenoside R_c which is the same as panaxoside D. The same compound isolated from American ginseng is also known as panaquilin C.[4] Confusing? Of course! So leave the details to the scientists and simply remember that whatever pharmacological activity ginseng may possess is probably due to its many chemical compounds which are triterpenoid saponins.

Obtaining the authentic ginseng product is a problem. Quality root is extremely expensive—the best grades of Korean Red (a specially "cured" root) retail at more than $20 an ounce. This relatively high cost plus lack of quality control in many areas of the "health food" industry have resulted in commercial ginseng products (teas, powders, capsules, tablets, extracts, etc.) of astounding variability. This has been verified by two independent studies,[7,8] one of which, an analysis of 54 ginseng products, showed that 60% of those analyzed were worthless and 25% of the sampled products contained no ginseng at all!

Another problem is the drug's relative safety. A study of 133 ginseng users seemed to point to a definite ginseng-abuse syndrome, especially in long-term users.[9] Some subjects taking this drug experienced high blood pressure, nervousness, and sleeplessness, while others had the opposite reactions, low blood pressure and a tranquilizing effect. Since the study included anything labeled "ginseng," even if quite different products such as canaigre were involved, these differences are not surprising. But taken as a whole, the symptoms of ginseng abuse were observed to mimic those of corticosteroid poisoning and serve to emphasize that if large amounts of ginseng are to be taken over an extended period, use caution!

Ginseng has also been reported to induce estrogen-like (female hormone-like) effects in women.[10] While certain changes of the vaginal mucosa may be desirable, the condition of mastalgia (painful breasts) with associated mammary nodularity (presence of nodules) is not. Vaginal bleeding has also been reported in a 72-year-old woman following consumption of ginseng. Such effects are attributed to the chemical similarity between the ginsenosides and the natural steroid hormones.

According to Siegel,[9] the term ginseng can refer to any of 22 different plants. Some of these are members of the same family (Araliaceae) or even genus (Panax). Others, such as canaigre, which are completely unrelated to ginseng either botanically or chemically, are downright frauds trading on the good reputation and high price of the original root. Two natural drugs which are closely enough related to ginseng botanically, chemically, and pharmacologically to be included here are so-called tienchi-ginseng and eleuthero.

Tienchi-ginseng, also known as tienchi, sanchi, or ginseng-sanchi, consists of the dried roots of Panax notoginseng (Burk.) F. H. Chen of the family Araliaceae. It is extensively cultivated in Yunnan Province, People's Republic of China. Analyses have shown that tienchi contains 7.0% to 10.8% of crude saponins in comparison to the approximately 4% found in normal oriental ginseng. Some of these saponins are identical to the ginsenosides found in the latter species.

In general, tienchi is used as a "tonic," but is recommended in particular for the prevention and treatment of coronary heart disease. No acute or short-term chronic toxicity was noted in small-animal tests; clinical studies in 680 cases of coronary disease also showed favorable outcomes.[11] The results of all these

Chinese studies require critical evaluation before the safety and efficacy of tienchi can be determined without question.

Eleuthero is not a species of *Panax* although it is a tall, prickly shrub of the same family, Araliaceae. The part used is the root of *Acanthopanax senticosus* (Rupr. et Maxim. ex Maxim.) Harms, which is more commonly referred to in the pharmaceutical literature as *Eleutherococcus senticosus* Maxim. This plant is native to eastern Siberia, Korea, and the Shansi and Hopei Provinces of China. The drug is also known as eleutherococc in the U.S.S.R., as Siberian ginseng in the United States, and as wujiaseng or ciwujia in China.

Although the constituents of eleuthero have been designated eleutherosides A through M, not all of these compounds are saponins of the types found in ginseng. Eleutheroside A, for example, is a β-sitosterol glycoside, and eleutheroside B_1 is a coumarin derivative.[12] Still, the same stimulant and tonic effects attributed to ginseng are also claimed for eleuthero. The Chinese report that its adaptogenic or antistress activity is brought about by the combination of contained sterols, coumarins, flavonoids, and polysaccharides.[13]

Large quantities of eleuthero originate in the Soviet Union, and at least part of its popularity as a ginseng substitute may derive from its abundance and relatively low cost, at least in comparison to original ginseng. Nevertheless, the same cautions noted for all of these saponin-containing drugs also apply to eleuthero. Lack of standardization of active principles, a potential abuse syndrome, and insufficiently tested clinical effects in human beings all speak against their indiscriminate use.[5]

Recently, Barna has aptly summarized the reasons why almost all of the biological studies thus far conducted on ginseng and related drugs stop with animal experimentation and are not carried further clinically in human subjects.[14] These include: (1) a lack of reliable, standardized ginseng preparations; (2) the near impossibility of obtaining patent protection for ginseng discoveries; (3) fundamental differences between Western and Oriental medicine; and (4) a lack of information on the proper dosage that is required to avoid side effects. As a result, he notes that only one well-controlled experiment with ginseng in human beings has ever been reported. Its results were equivocal. Until additional clinical studies are conducted and their results are reported and analyzed, it is necessary to agree with Lewis' conclusion regarding this interesting herb:[15] "Unfortunately, ginseng remains a medical enigma with no proven efficacy for humans."

REFERENCES

1. Abstracts of Korean Ginseng Studies (1687–1975), The Research Institute, Office of Monopoly, Republic of Korea, 1975.
2. L. H. Bailey and E. Z. Bailey: Hortus Third. Macmillan, New York, 1976, p. 815.
3. N. R. Farnsworth: Tile & Till 59: 30–32, 1973.
4. J. P. Hou: The Myth and Truth About Ginseng. A. S. Barnes and Co., South Brunswick, N.J., 1978.
5. V. E. Tyler, L. R. Brady, and J. E. Robbers: Pharmacognosy, 8th Ed. Lea & Febiger, Philadelphia, 1981, pp. 481–484.
6. A. Y. Leung: Encyclopedia of Common Natural Ingredients Used in Food, Drugs, and Cosmetics. John Wiley & Sons, New York, 1980, pp. 186–189.
7. L. E. Liberti and A. Der Marderosian: Journal of Pharmaceutical Sciences 67: 1487–1489, 1978.
8. W. Ziglar: Whole Foods 2(4): 48–53, 1979.
9. R. K. Siegel: Journal of the American Medical Association 241: 1614–1615, 1979; 243: 32, 1980.
10. Anon.: Lawrence Review of Natural Products 6(9): not pgd., 1985.
11. Tienchi-Ginseng, China National Native Produce & Animal By-Products Import & Export Corp., Yunnan Native Produce Branch, Kunming, 1979, not pgd.
12. J. Connert: Deutsche Apotheker Zeitung 120: 735–736, 1980.
13. Wujiaseng, China National Native Produce & Animal By-Products Import & Export Corp., Heilungkiang Native Produce Branch, n.d., not pgd.
14. P. Barna: Lancet II: 548, 1985.
15. W. Lewis: *In* Plants in Indigenous Medicine & Diet: Behavioral Approaches, N. L. Etkin, Ed. Redgrave Publishing Co., Bedford Hills, N.Y., 1986, pp. 290–305.

GOLDENSEAL

oldenseal or hydrastis is a native American drug, having been introduced to the early settlers by the Cherokee Indians who used it primarily for skin diseases and as a wash for sore eyes. It consists of the rhizome and roots of the small forest plant *Hydrastis canadensis* L., a member of the family Ranunculaceae.[1] Over the years, goldenseal acquired a considerable reputation as a general bitter tonic and as a remedy for various gastric and genitourinary disorders. The drug was a prominent ingredient in many turn-of-the-century proprietary medicines, including Dr. Pierce's Golden Medical Discovery.

> *A few of my symptoms were: Heartburn and fullness after eating, sometimes pain in my bowels, headache, poor appetite, and bad taste in my mouth. At night I was feverish, with hot flushes over my skin. After taking Dr. Pierce's Golden Medical Discovery I was relieved of all these symptoms, and I feel perfectly well today.*

> J. P. McAdams
> Elon College, North Carolina[2]

Whatever activity is possessed by goldenseal can be attributed to its contained alkaloids, especially hydrastine and berberine. The latter is also responsible for the drug's characteristic golden color. While these alkaloids, and consequently the whole drug, do exert some minor actions on circulation, uterine tone and contractility, and on the central nervous system, unless extremely large, near-toxic doses are administered, the effects are too uncertain to be therapeutically useful. Goldenseal is no longer even discussed in modern works on pharmacology, and Sollmann[3] has concluded that it "has few, if any, rational indications." Nevertheless, it continues to occupy a place of prominence in modern herbals; one of them devotes 78 pages to a discussion of the various aspects of this interesting drug.[4]

A recent survey of folk medicine in Indiana produced so many endorsements of goldenseal tea as a useful rinse to relieve sore mouth, cracked and bleeding lips, canker sores, and related problems, that this use must at least be mentioned here.[5] The previously mentioned alkaloids do possess both astringent and weak antiseptic properties which cause goldenseal tea to be a modestly effective local treatment in many such cases.

Several years ago, goldenseal gained considerable publicity from the claim that usually as an herbal tea, it prevented the detection of morphine in urine specimens following heroin use. It thus achieved considerable popularity among certain heroin addicts who were patients in methadone or similar drug rehabilitation programs. Scientific studies have revealed no basis for this claim. Goldenseal neither prevents morphine detection nor does it "flush" that compound from the body.[6] Nevertheless, this myth continues to exist in expanded form in the late 1980's. Personnel in "health food" stores and head shops (stores specializing in drug-abuse paraphernalia) on the West Coast are reported to be recommending the consumption of goldenseal as a means of thwarting the now widely used urine tests designed to detect illegal use of marihuana and/or cocaine. Authorities, however, disagree:[7] As *High Times* has repeatedly warned, *no* edible substance, taken internally, will have any effect at all on drug-urinalysis machines (except to possibly promote *false-positive* readings).

REFERENCES

1. V. E. Tyler, L. R. Brady, and J. E. Robbers: Pharmacognosy, 8th Ed. Lea & Febiger, Philadelphia, 1981, p. 223, 485.
2. R. V. Pierce: The People's Common Sense Medical Adviser, 62nd Ed. World's Dispensary Printing Office and Bindery, Buffalo, N.Y., 1895, p. 589.
3. T. Sollmann: A Manual of Pharmacology, 7th Ed. W. B. Saunders, Philadelphia, 1948, pp. 257–258.
4. L. Veninga and B. R. Zaricor: Goldenseal/Etc., Ruka Publications, Santa Cruz, Calif., 1976, pp. 1–78.
5. V. E. Tyler: Hoosier Home Remedies. Purdue University Press, West Lafayette, Indiana, 1985, pp. 138–139.
6. J. A. Ostrenga and D. Perry: PharmChem Newsletter 4(1): 1–3, 1975.
7. M. W. Montague: High Times No. 135: 15, 85, 93, 1986.

GOTU KOLA

"Two leaves a day will keep old age away."
                    Ancient Sinhalese Proverb

The leaves in this saying are those of *Centella asiatica* (L.) Urb. (family Umbelliferae), a slender creeping plant which is especially abundant in the swampy areas of India and Sri Lanka, South Africa, and the tropical regions of the New World. It is commonly called gotu kola but is also known as hydrocotyle or Indian pennywort.

In Sri Lanka, it was observed that elephants, noted for their longevity among beasts, fed extensively on the plant. This gave rise to the reputation of the herb as a longevity promoter. Eating a few leaves daily was thought to "strengthen and revitalize worn out bodies and brains." Gotu kola has also been recommended as a treatment for mental troubles, high blood pressure, abscesses, rheumatism, fever, ulcers, leprosy, skin eruptions, nervous disorders, and jaundice.[1] More recently, the drug has acquired a considerable reputation as an aphrodisiac, an agent which stimulates sexual desire and ability.[2]

Scientific studies have shown that in relatively large doses the drug has a definite sedative effect in small animals. This activity comes from two saponin glycosides designated brahmoside and brahminoside.[3] Another glycoside, known as madecassoside, exhibits some anti-inflammatory activity and still another, asiaticoside, apparently stimulates wound healing.[4] However, there is currently no evidence to support the use of gotu kola as a longevity promoter or to substantiate any of the other extravagant claims made for it as a revitalizing and healing herb. Substantive data on its safety and efficacy are simply nonexistent.

A word of caution is necessary about the name of this herb. The similarity in spelling has caused gotu kola to be confused with the dried cotyledon (seed leaf) of *Cola nitida* (Vent.) Schott et Endl., otherwise known as kolanuts, kola, or cola.[5] This plant material, well-known as an ingredient of Coca-Cola®, contains up to 3.5% of caffeine, a constituent not present in gotu kola. Whatever else it may be, gotu kola is certainly not a stimulant.

REFERENCES

1. V. De Silva: Medical Herbalist 11: 159, 1936.
2. A. Gottlieb: Sex Drugs and Aphrodisiacs, High Times/Level Press, New York and San Francisco, 1974, pp. 37–38.
3. A. S. Ramaswamy, S. M. Periyasamy, and N. Basu: Journal of Research in Indian Medicine 4: 160–175, 1970.
4. P. H. List and L. Hörhammer, Eds.: Hagers Handbuch der Pharmazeutischen Praxis, 4th Ed. Vol.. 3. Springer-Verlag, Berlin, 1972, pp. 792–793.
5. R. K. Siegel: Journal of the American Medical Association 236: 473–476, 1976.

HAWTHORN

Although some of the medicinal properties of the fruits or haws of this small- to medium-sized tree, *Crataegus oxycantha* L. (family Rosaceae), were known to Dioscorides in the first century A.D., and the drug continued to be mentioned by Gerard and other early herbalists, hawthorn was not widely used therapeutically until very recent times.[1] Even now, the drug, which may be obtained from several closely related *Crataegus* species, is little known in the United States. But hawthorn flowers, fruits, and leaves are prominent in Continental medicine. About three dozen different preparations containing extracts of these plant parts, either singly or in combination with other drugs, are currently marketed in Germany. That figure does not include a number of herbal mixtures or teas which have hawthorn as one of their major ingredients.

However, this interesting plant has not been entirely neglected, even in this country. A 125-page book titled *The Hawthorn Berry for the Heart*, devoted to a discussion of its medicinal properties, was published in 1971.[2] Hawthorn is described in it and most other modern herbals[3-5] as a valuable drug for the treatment of various heart ailments and circulatory disorders. Wrongly believing that only the bark contained cardioactive principles, Gibbons experimented with haw jelly and haw marmalade, even giving some to his friends at Christmas.[6] He described these daily astringent products as a very pleasant way of treating a sore throat. Since the haws, leaves, and flowers all contain compounds which do affect the heart and circulatory system, products containing them should not be consumed indiscriminately. Interestingly, it was not until 1974, some years after Gibbons made his comments, that a scientific study revealed that the bark of a *Crataegus* species contained any active principles.[7]

Modern research has revealed some interesting properties of hawthorn. It acts on the body in two ways: First, it dilates the blood vessels, especially the coronary vessels, reducing peripheral resistance and thus lowering the blood pressure. It is thought to reduce the tendency to angina attacks. Second, it apparently has a direct, favorable effect on the heart itself which is especially noticeable in cases of heart damage. Hawthorn's action is not immediate but develops very slowly. Its toxicity is low as well, becoming evident only in large doses. It therefore seems to be a relatively harmless, mild heart tonic which apparently yields good results in many conditions where this kind of therapy is required.[1]

The active principles of hawthorn are probably a mixture of pigments known as flavonoids, large numbers of which are contained in the various plant parts. So-called oligomeric procyanidins (dehydrocatechins) seem to be particularly active.[8] They also produce marked sedative effects which indicate an action on the central nervous system.

Further scientific studies may eventually substantiate these findings; in fact, studies are urgently needed for a drug as potentially valuable as this one. Until additional research has been carried out, prospective users of hawthorn for heart and circulation problems should consider all the consequences. Users of self-selected medicines almost always do so as a result of self-diagnosis. This is a very dangerous practice when such vital systems of the human body as the heart and blood vessels are involved. For this reason, self-treatment with hawthorn is neither advocated nor condoned.

REFERENCES

1. E. Steinegger and R. Hänsel: Lehrbuch der Pharmakognosie, 3rd Ed. Springer-Verlag, Berlin, 1972, pp. 146–147.
2. J. I. Rodale: The Hawthorn Berry for the Heart. Rodale Books, Emmaus, Pa., 1971.
3. D. Law: The Concise Herbal Encyclopedia. Saint Martin's Press, New York, 1973, pp. 56–57; 116.
4. R. Lucas: Nature's Medicines. Wilshire Book Co., North Hollywood, Calif., 1977, pp. 188–189.
5. M. Tierra: The Way of Herbs. Unity Press, Santa Cruz, Calif., 1980., p. 97.
6. E. Gibbons: Stalking the Healthful Herbs, Field Guide Ed. David McKay Co., New York, 1970, pp. 171–174.
7. E. B. Thompson, G. H. Aynilian, P. Gora, and N. R. Farnsworth: Journal of Pharmaceutical Sciences 63: 1936–1937, 1974.
8. W. Rewerski, T. Piechocki, M. Rylski, and S. Lewak: Arzneimittel-Forschung 21: 886–888, 1971.

HIBISCUS

A variety of names — hibiscus, roselle, Sudanese tea, red tea, and Jamaica sorrel — designate the flowers (actually calyx and bracts) of *Hibiscus sabdariffa* L. This red-flowered annual herb of the family Malvaceae is widely cultivated throughout the tropics, reaching a height of 4 to 5 feet or more. Its flower heads are collected when immature and are highly prized for making jams, jellies, sauces, and acid beverages.[1] The floral parts make a pleasant tea and are used by themselves or mixed with other herb teas.[2]

Hibiscus contains various anthocyanins and other pigments plus relatively large amounts of oxalic, malic, citric (12% to 17%), and tartaric acid, as well as up to 28% of hibiscic acid (the lactone of a hydroxycitric acid).[3] These plant acids are responsible for the tart, refreshing taste of various hibiscus beverages and foods. They probably also account for the mild laxative and diuretic effects attributed to the plant.

Reports of other physiological properties of hibiscus are insubstantial and require verification. For example, its hypotensive (blood-pressure lowering) action was observed only on direct injection of an extract into the vein of a dog; the effect was very brief, even when large amounts were given.[4] Critical reevaluation of the experiments in which hibiscus extracts were found to inhibit the growth of the tubercle bacillus is also advisable.[5]

Widely employed throughout the world as a beverage and food flavor, hibiscus imparts a taste which is obviously pleasant to many people. So there appears to be no reason to discourage anyone from using it for this purpose.

REFERENCES

1. L. H. Bailey and E. Z. Bailey: Hortus Third. Macmillan, New York, 1976, pp. 562, 982–983.
2. M. Stuart, Ed.: The Encyclopedia of Herbs and Herbalism, Grosset & Dunlap, New York, 1979, p. 201.
3. A. Y. Leung: Encyclopedia of Common Natural Ingredients Used in Food, Drugs, and Cosmetics, John Wiley & Sons, New York, 1980, pp. 282–283.
4. A. Sharaf: Planta Medica 10: 48–52, 1962.
5. A. Sharaf and A. Gineidi: Ibid 11: 109–112, 1963.

HONEY

Honey is the saccharine secretion deposited in the honeycomb by the bee, *Apis mellifera* L., a well-known insect of the family Apidae. To prepare this product, the worker bee collects nectar from various flowers and stores it briefly in its crop or honey-bag. There it is acted upon by secretions from glands in the bee's head and thorax which bring about various changes, particularly conversion of much of the contained sucrose (cane sugar) to so-called invert or simple sugars. On returning to the hive, the insect regurgitates the viscous liquid, now known as honey, into the wax comb where it is extracted for marketing.[1]

The 1811 edition of The Edinburgh New Dispensatory[2] informs us that, "From the earliest ages, honey has been employed as a medicine . . . it forms an excellent gargle and facilitates the expectoration of viscid phlegm; and it is sometimes employed as an emollient application to abscesses, and as a detergent to ulcers." More recent advocates of the medicinal use of honey have greatly expanded its purported virtues. D. C. Jarvis, a Vermont physician who advocated a mixture of honey and vinegar as a cure-all, has written a detailed account of the so-called therapeutic uses of honey. He claimed that it improved digestion; attracted fluid and thereby facilitated the healing of wounds and ulcers; helped the body destroy harmful germs; was an excellent food supplement because of its content of vitamins, minerals, and enzymes; was a useful laxative; had a sedative effect; and helped to relieve arthritis pain. As if these seven actions were not sufficient, he also maintained that persons who ate honey and kept bees were entirely free from cancer and paralysis.[3]

Because of its commercial importance as a nutrient and sweetener, honey has been subjected to extensive chemical analyses. It consists of about 40% fructose (fruit sugar), 35% glucose (grape sugar), 4% other sugars including sucrose, 18% water, and 3% other substances such as aromatic principles and tannin. Vitamins, minerals, and proteins (enzymes) are also present but in such tiny amounts as to preclude any therapeutic utility or, for that matter, any real nutritional significance.[4]

Of course, honey is a tasty and useful sweetening agent; it serves as a rapid source of energy because it contains simple sugars. Honey also is still used in folk medicine for its demulcent or soothing effects, particularly in various cough remedies. However, there is no evidence to support claims of any sedative action or that it will relieve the pain of arthritis or any other affliction. References to its role in preventing or curing cancer or paralysis are gross exaggerations. Whatever antibacterial properties honey may possess are due primarily to its high sugar content. Once, diluted by contact with body or other fluids, any such effect is lost.

Like the queen in the Mother Goose rhyme, I do savor the taste of honey:

> "The queen was in the parlor,
> Eating bread and honey."

It is an elegant spread for bread or rolls. Honey added to hot lemonade effectively soothes a sore throat and may, in one way or another, even help ease the cold which caused it. Beyond this, it is unrealistic to expect any significant medicinal value from the product. Your expectations simply will not be realized.

REFERENCES

1. H. W. Felter and J. U. Lloyd: King's American Dispensatory, 18th Ed., Vol. 2. The Ohio Valley Co., Cincinnati, 1900, pp. 1247–1249.
2. A. Duncan, Jr.: The Edinburgh New Dispensatory, 6th Ed. Bell & Bradfute, Edinburgh, 1811, pp. 324–325.
3. D. C. Jarvis: Arthritis and Folk Medicine, Reprint Ed. Fawcett Publications, Greenwich, Conn., 1960, pp. 134–137.
4. D. Johnson: In Whole Foods Natural Foods Guide, And/Or Press, Berkeley, Calif., 1979, pp. 76–79.

HOPS

The hop plant, *Humulus lupulus* L., a member of the family Moraceae, is a perennial climbing vine which bears scaly cone-like fruits known as hops. These fruits, technically called strobiles, are covered with glandular hairs containing resinous bitter principles which account for the use of hops in brewing and in medicine. Hops are extensively cultivated in England, Germany, the United States, South America, and Australia. They are collected in September when ripe and marketed after careful drying.[1]

Although hops have been used in beer primarily for their bitter taste and preservative action for over 1000 years, their medicinal or tonic properties were apparently also valued from very early times. It was observed that hop pickers tired easily, apparently as a result of the accidental transfer of some hop resin from their hands to their mouths, and the drug gained a reputation as a sedative. Pillows filled with hops have been used for sleeplessness and nervous conditions. A small bag of hops, wetted with alcohol and placed hot on the afflicted area was said to reduce local inflammation. Aqueous extracts made with boiling water have been used as tonics.

"TAKE HOP BITTERS three times a day, and you will have no doctor bills to pay," was the advertising slogan of one patent medicine manufacturer in the last century. In addition to hops, this popular product contained some buchu, mandrake, dandelion, and 30% alcohol. During the 4-year period preceding 1884, $2.75 million worth of this nostrum was sold.[2]

Chemically unstable polyphenolic principles, especially humulone and lupulone, are present in the resin of hops. They, or closely related conversion products, are responsible for the plant's bitter and bacteriostatic properties. Unfortunately, the content of these compounds varies appreciably in different varieties of hops and besides, they are quite unstable in the presence of air and light. One study has shown that after nine months' storage, hops retained only about 15% of their original activity.[3]

Early studies on hops failed to identify specific sedative principles, and their value, particularly when used in the form of a pillow, was thought to be more magical than medicinal. More recently, a volatile alcohol, 2-methyl-3-butene-2-ol, has been isolated from hops and is believed to account for at least part of the plant's sedative properties.[4] Present in fresh hops in very small amounts, the concentration of the alcohol increases on drying to reach a maximum value of about 0.15% within a 2-year period.

Mobility tests in rats verified the sedative-hypnotic activity of the alcohol, and pharmacologically active concentrations of it were detected in freshly prepared hop teas. Although studies thus far carried out do not provide an explanation for all of the salutary effects attributed to hops by folklore, they do supply, for the first time, a logical scientific basis for at least part of their tranquilizing action. Continuing investigations will probably eventually supply the rest of the story regarding their benefit to mankind.

Hops are closely related botanically to marihuana, and some writers advocate smoking the plant material to obtain a mild euphoria.[5] This practice cannot be recommended since unpleasant side effects are common, and the safety of smoking hops remains in doubt.

REFERENCES

1. V. E. Tyler, L. R. Brady, and J. E. Robbers: Pharmacognosy, 8th Ed. Lea & Febiger, Philadelphia, 1981, pp. 486–487.
2. H. W. Holcombe: Patent Medicine Tax Stamps. Quaterman Publications, Lawrence, Mass., 1979, pp. 248–251.
3. G. Berndt: Deutsche Apotheker-Zeitung 106: 158–159, 1966.
4. R. Wohlfart: Deutsche Apotheker-Zeitung 123: 1637–1638, 1983.
5. L. A. Young, L. G. Young, M. M. Klein, D. M. Klein, and D. Beyer: Recreational Drugs. Collier Books, New York, 1977, p. 98.

HOREHOUND

Horehound or hoarhound is a hairy, bitter-aromatic, perennial herb native to the Mediterranean region of Europe and Asia but naturalized in North America. Designated botanically as *Marrubium vulgare* L. and classified in the mint family or Labiatae, its leaves and flowering tops have long been widely used, both as a folk medicine and a flavoring agent. The common name, horehound, derives from the abundant whitish hairs which cover the plant's leaves, giving them a hoary appearance; hound refers to the use of the plant by the ancient Greeks to treat mad-dog bite.

Nearly four centuries ago, Gerard praised horehound's usefulness in treating coughs and consumption (tuberculosis), and more recently Grieve noted its expectorant, tonic, and antiasthmatic properties.[1] It is also said to act as a stomachic, a vermifuge, and in large doses, a purgative. Applied externally, it is recommended as a treatment for wounds. Probably the most common use of horehound today is in lozenges and syrups intended for the relief of coughs and minor throat irritations. Most children today are familiar with the taste of horehound candy.

References attribute the activity of the herb to a combination of marrubiin, a bitter diterpenoid lactone principle which has been isolated from it in concentrations ranging from 0.3 to 1.0%; volatile oil; and tannin. However, marrubiin is now known to be an artifact which does not preexist in the plant but is formed from the closely related premarrubiin during the isolation procedure.[2]

Horehound is apparently an effective expectorant. This property is a result, not so much of the contained volatile oil, but of the marrubiin (premarrubiin) which stimulates the secretions of the bronchial mucosa.[3] Other pharmacological effects attributed to the drug are more problematical and require extensive investigation before they can be judged either significant or useful. Marrubiin is reputed to be effective in normalizing cardiac arrhythmias (heart irregularities) — but in large doses can *cause* them. Marrubic acid, which can be formed from marrubiin, has been shown to stimulate the flow of bile in rats.[4] This might account for the purgative properties observed with large doses, but it is really difficult to evaluate since the marrubic acid content of horehound is unknown.

The pleasant fragrance and taste of horehound volatile oil plus the expectorant action of its bitter principle account for the widespread use of the herb and its extracts for coughs and colds. This appears to be the only use for this ancient folk medicine which can presently be justified.

REFERENCES

1. M. Grieve: A Modern Herbal, Vol. 1. Dover Publications, New York, 1971, pp. 415–416.
2. M. S. Henderson and R. McCrindle: Journal of the Chemical Society, Section C: 1969, 2014–2015.
3. P. H. List and L. Hörhammer, Eds.: Hagers Handbuch der Pharmazeutischen Praxis, 4th Ed., Vol. 5. Springer-Verlag, Berlin, 1976, pp. 703–706.
4. I. Krejčí and R. Zadina: Planta Medica 7: 1–7, 1959.

HORSETAIL

Art's perfect forms no moral need,
And beauty is its own excuse;
But for the dull and flowerless weed
Some healing virtue still must plead.
John Greenleaf Whittier
Songs of Labor, Dedication, Stanza 5

There are those who plead eloquently for the healing virtues of the "dull and flowerless weed" known as horsetail. *Equisetum arvense* L. (family Equisetaceae) is technically a pteridophyte and thus is more closely related to the ferns than to the flowering plants. Horsetail is a rush-like perennial with hollow, jointed stems and scale-like leaves, reproducing by means of spores, not seeds. The stems contain large amounts of silica and silicic acids (5–8%) which account for its use as a metal polisher and its synonym of souring rush. Several closely related species of *Equisetum* are similar to *E. arvense* in appearance and use.

Enthusiasts call horsetail a valuable diuretic and astringent for treating various kidney and bladder ailments ranging from kidney stones to cystic ulceration, and also recommend it as a rapid-acting remedy for dropsy. It is also called effective in treating tuberculosis, especially when accompanied by the "spitting of blood." External application is supposed to stop the bleeding of wounds and promote rapid healing.[1,2]

In addition to the silica compounds, horsetail contains about 5% of a saponin designated equisetonin and several flavone glycosides including isoquercitrin, galuteolin, and equisetrin.[3] A very small amount of nicotine (0.00004%) is also present.[4] The flavone glycosides and the saponin probably combine to account for the diuretic action of horsetail which has been demonstrated experimentally but which is very slight.[5] There is no valid experimental evidence to support the hypothesis that the silica and silicic acid derivatives in the drug promote the healing of bleeding tubercular lesions in the lung.[6]

Even vigorous pleading does not produce much scientific support for the healing virtues of horsetail. The plant is a weak diuretic and little else.

REFERENCES

1. M. Grieve: A Modern Herbal, Vol. 1. Dover Publications, New York, 1971, pp. 419–421.
2. H. Kreitmair: Die Pharmazie 8: 298–300, 1953.
3. H. A. Hoppe: Drogenkunde, 8th Ed., Vol. 2. Walter de Gruyter, Berlin, 1977, pp. 173–176.
4. J. D. Phillipson and C. Melville: Journal of Pharmacy and Pharmacology 12: 506–508, 1960.
5. H. Vollmer and K. Hübner: Naunyn-Schmiedebergs Archiv für experimentelle Pathologie und Pharmakologie 186: 565–573, 592–605, 1937.
6. E. Steinegger and R. Hänsel: Lehrbuch der Pharmakognosie, 3rd Ed. Springer-Verlag, Berlin, 1972, p. 214.

HYDRANGEA

Hydrangea or seven barks consists of the underground portions (rhizome and roots) of the plant *Hydrangea arborescens* L. (family Saxifragaceae), an erect shrub growing in the eastern part of the United States from New York to Florida and west to Oklahoma.[1] It was originally used by the Cherokee Indians who introduced it to the early settlers as a remedy for kidney stones. During the first few decades of this century, the drug saw some action for this and also as a diuretic in conventional medicine, but it lapsed into disuse until the recent revival of herbal remedies. Advocates of herbal medicine still recommend it for these conditions.[2]

There is no evidence, aside from empirical observations and anecdotes, that hydrangea has any therapeutic utility at all. But then, there have been no modern scientific studies of the drug's physiological activity and practically no investigations of its chemistry.[3] For example, a crystalline compound first isolated in 1887 and designated hydrangin remains chemically unidentified nearly 100 years later.

Hydrangea would probably not merit being included in this book—for there are certainly more effective diuretics and treatments for kidney stones—if it were not for the publicity surrounding another species of the same genus. The hydrangea ordinarily cultivated for its showy flowers is *Hydrangea paniculata* Siebold, particularly a cultivar of that species designated Grandiflora. Its leaves have been smoked in a fashion analogous to marihuana to produce a kind of euphoria or "high." However, even the books devoted to such intoxicants emphasize that this practice "will either get one very stoned or very sick," as a result of a cyanide-producing compound contained in the leaves.[4]

There is no question that the practice can make the user very sick, but there is some doubt that the poisonous character of the leaves is due to cyanide. Reports dating back to the early 1900's did detect cyanide-producing compounds in the leaves of certain *Hydrangea* species, but the common ornamental variety was not among them. Hegnauer has concluded that probably only a few members of the genus may have this property and then in significant amounts only during the early stages of vegetative development.[5]

Still, the questionable identity of the toxic principle does not make smoking hydrangea leaves any more advisable or the illness which can result from it any less real. As a drug of use or abuse, the roots or leaves of any *Hydrangea* species have no merit except for the weak diuretic action of the underground parts of *H. arborescens.*

REFERENCES

1. H. W. Felter and J. U. Lloyd: King's American Dispensatory, Vol 2. The Ohio Valley Co., Cincinnati, 1900, pp. 1000–1001.
2. N. Coon: Using Plants for Healing, 2nd Ed. Rodale Press, Emmaus, Pa., 1979, p. 122.
3. A. Y. Leung: Encyclopedia of Common Natural Ingredients Used in Food, Drugs, and Cosmetics. John Wiley & Sons, New York, 1980, pp. 201–202.
4. L. A. Young, L. G. Young, M. M. Klein, D. M. Klein, and D. Beyer: Recreational Drugs, Collier Books, New York, 1977, p. 99.
5. R. Hegnauer: Chemotaxonomie der Pflanzen, Vol. 6. Birkhäuser Verlag, Basel, 1973, p. 326.

HYSSOP

Almost all the write-ups on this plant in modern herbals include a few choice biblical quotations referring to its ritualistic use in cleansing people or places.[1-3] These quotations are extremely misleading, for it is very doubtful if the well-known garden herb *Hyssopus officinalis* L. which is now called "hyssop" has any relation whatever to the plant mentioned in the Old and New Testaments. Learned discussions regarding the identity of the biblical hyssop were underway some 250 years ago, and even then, more than 18 different plants had been suggested.[4] The plant's true identity will probably never be established.

Even in the 20th century, considerable confusion exists about the name hyssop. Therefore, we must affirm again that the plant discussed here under that title is just plain hyssop (*Hyssopus officinalis* L.) and not giant hyssop, hedge hyssop, prairie hyssop, or wild hyssop, all of which are entirely different species.

Hyssop is a perennial shrub of the family Labiatae which has been naturalized in the United States. It is a common garden plant which also grows widely along the sides of roads. As is the case with many other mints, its leaves contain an appreciable amount of volatile oil, giving them a camphor-like odor and a somewhat bitter taste. This volatile oil is an ingredient in many French liqueurs, specifically those which resemble Chartreuse and Benedictine.[5] It is also the agent responsible for the household medicinal use of the plant, mostly as tea, for coughs, colds, hoarseness, fevers, and sore throats.[2] Hyssop tea, mixed with a little honey, is said to be especially effective as an expectorant (an agent which promotes the loosening and expulsion of phlegm).

Because of the presence of pinocamphone, isopinocamphone, α- and β-pinene, camphene, and α-terpinene, which together make up about 70% of the oil,[6] hyssop is a reasonably effective treatment for mild irritations of the respiratory tract that accompany the common cold. It is also generally recognized as safe; no adverse reports of its safety appear in the scientific literature.

On the other hand, claims of its ability to treat wounds or cuts (even those made with rusty farm implements) because the mold that produces penicillin grows on hyssop leaves, must be regarded as so much nonsense.[7] *Penicillium* species are among the most ubiquitous of fungi and grow anywhere there are sufficient moisture, nutrients, and a suitable temperature. It is highly unlikely that the sparse growths occurring on hyssop leaves would produce any viable amount of antibiotic. Any antiseptic action of the leaves would more likely be due to its volatile oil. Such an effect would be relatively weak at best and would certainly not be significant in the treatment of puncture wounds susceptible to tetanus (lockjaw) infection.

REFERENCES

1. R. Lucas: Nature's Medicines, Wilshire Book Co., North Hollywood, Calif., 1977, p. 25.
2. W. H. Hylton, Ed.: The Rodale Herb Book, Rodale Press Book Div., Emmaus, Pa., 1976, pp. 474–478.
3. R. C. Wren and R. W. Wren: Potter's New Cyclopaedia of Botanical Drugs and Herbs, New Health Science Press, Hengiscote, England, 1975, p. 160.
4. H. N. Moldenke and A. L. Moldenke: Plants of the Bible. Chronica Botanica Company, Waltham, Mass., 1952, pp. 160–162.
5. E. Guenther: The Essential Oils, Vol. 3. D. Van Nostrand Company, New York, 1949, pp. 436–440.
6. A. Y. Leung: Encyclopedia of Common Natural Ingredients Used in Food, Drugs, and Cosmetics. John Wiley & Sons, New York, 1980, pp. 202–203.
7. D. Hall: The Book of Herbs. Charles Scribner's Sons, New York, 1972, pp. 126–129.

JOJOBA OIL

It is difficult to pick up a newspaper or magazine nowadays without finding at least one advertisement for some kind of jojoba (pronounced hohóba) oil cosmetic preparation. Shampoos are most common, but various kinds of creams and lotions containing the "rare oil used by American Indians for hundreds of years as a cosmetic and medicinal aid" are also offered. Yet even knowledgeable people have had difficulty in differentiating jojoba from Ho! Ho! Ho! or even Ho Chi Minh! Just what is this mysterious substance which seems to be so popular of late?

Jojoba wax (technically it is not an oil) is obtained from the peanut-sized seeds of the jojoba plant, *Simmondsia chinensis* (Link) C. K. Schneid., also referred to as *S. californica* (Link) Nutt. This evergreen shrub of the family Buxaceae grows in abundance on rocky desert hillsides in Arizona, California, and Mexico. Commonly called goat nuts, the seeds of the plant resemble coffee beans. When expressed, they yield about 50% of a liquid wax, composed almost entirely of high molecular weight, monoethylenic acids (eicosenoic acid — 35%) and alcohols (eicosenol — 22%, docosenol — 21%). The wax, known commonly as jojoba oil, in its physical properties resembles sperm oil[1] formerly obtained from the sperm whale (now an endangered species). It may be hydrogenated to produce a solid wax that is similar to spermaceti.

The American Indians reportedly used the oil as a hair dressing. Now it is incorporated into jojoba oil shampoos considered especially effective in preventing the buildup of sebum (the fatty material secreted by sebacous glands) on the scalp. The reasoning behind this theory is that jojoba oil resembles sebum in many respects, both chemically and physically. By coating the scalp with jojoba oil, it is believed (but not proven) that the natural production of sebum will be reduced.[2] Of course, whether it is more desirable to have the scalp coated with jojoba oil or with sebum is a moot question. The oil is readily taken up by the skin and imparts a velvety softness to it and to the hair as well. This lubrication of the scalp does, no doubt, reduce the flaking of the skin normally associated with dandruff.

Overly enthusiastic advocates of jojoba oil, known in the trade as "jojoba witnesses," tout the product for restoring lost hair and preventing further hair loss, for removing warts, curing cancer, and other similar uses. Needless to say, there is absolutely no scientific evidence to support such claims.

Toxicity tests on jojoba oil for external application have caused no significant concern. Aside from causing occasional allergic responses in sensitive individuals, the product may be considered safe for human skin.[3] Whether the various preparations containing this unusual liquid wax are any more effective than similar cosmetics containing the customary emollient oils is something which will be very difficult to prove scientifically. As with most such products, this is best judged subjectively by each user.

REFERENCES

1. A. H. Warth: The Chemistry and Technology of Wax. Rheinhold Publishing Corp., New York, 1947, pp. 172–176.
2. T. K. Miwa: Cosmetics and Perfumery 88: 39–41, 1973.
3. J. H. Brown: Manufacturing Chemist and Aerosol News 50(6): 47, 1979.

JUNIPER

Persons of legal age who are not familiar with the odor and taste of juniper have led sheltered lives. For well over 300 years, gin has been one of the most popular alcoholic beverages of the Western world, most of whose inhabitants have some familiarity with the dry martini or other juniper-flavored concoctions. The fleshy, purplish fruits (berries) of *Juniperus communis* L., an evergreen shrub or small tree of the family Cupressaceae, contain 0.2% to 2% of a volatile oil which is the principal flavoring agent in gin.

Juniper and its volatile oil have long enjoyed a considerable reputation in folk medicine as a diuretic and as a treatment in various conditions of the kidneys and bladder. They are also recommended for their carminative action in cases of indigestion and flatulence.[1] The berries are usually taken in the form of a tea prepared from juniper in a mixture with other drugs, but for treating rheumatism, the berries themselves are eaten. The berries are also said to have a stimulating effect on the appetite; this may account for their incorporation as a flavoring agent in such dishes as sauerkraut. Extracting the berries with 70% alcohol yields a volatile oil-rich preparation, technically called a "spirit," which is suggested for either external or internal use in these conditions.[2]

The diuretic action of juniper results from its contained volatile oil and specifically the constituent designated terpinen-4-ol which increases the glomerular filtration rate in the kidneys.[3] However, excessive doses of the drug may produce kidney irritation, and in the case of persons already suffering from kidney disease, this can result from even normal therapeutic doses. Juniper and its preparations must not be used by expectant mothers since they not only increase intestinal movements but also stimulate contraction of the uterus.[4] The concentration of juniper oil in commercial alcoholic beverages is quite small, not exceeding 0.006%,[5] so imbibers should not expect therapeutic responses when these are consumed (at least in reasonable amounts).

Because it acts as a diuretic by causing local irritation of the kidneys—and because this action is liable to be detrimental when those organs are already inflamed—and because juniper is hazardous for use by pregnant mothers, this drug is no longer recommended for various kidney disorders by the medical profession. Safer and much more effective drugs certainly exist, but juniper continues to be used in folk medicine, particularly for its diuretic properties.

REFERENCES

1. M. Grieve: A Modern Herbal, Vol. 2. Dover Publications, New York, 1971, pp. 452–453.
2. M. Pahlow: Das grosse Buch der Heilpflanzen, Gräfe und Unzer GmbH, Munich, 1979, pp. 341–342.
3. J. Janku, M. Hava, and O. Motl: Experientia 13: 255–256, 1957.
4. P. H. List and L. Hörhammer, Eds.: Hagers Handbuch der Pharmazeutischen Praxis, 4th Ed., Vol. 5. Springer-Verlag, Berlin, 1976, pp. 333–337.
5. A. Y. Leung: Encyclopedia of Common Natural Ingredients Used in Food, Drugs, and Cosmetics, John Wiley & Sons, New York, 1980, pp. 208–209.

KELP

Kelp is such an imprecise generic term that no two authorities seem to agree on the identity of the plant(s) it supposedly designates. Definitions range all the way from a single species, *Fucus vesiculosus* L.[1] to any kind of coarse seaweeds, or more precisely, the ash obtained by burning them.[2] In modern times, kelp most probably refers to seaweeds of the brown algal order Laminariales which possess large, flat, leaflike fronds, especially species of *Laminaria, Macrocystis,* and *Nereocystis.*[3] This definition should be broadened, however, to include several species of another order, Fucales or rockweed, since several authors indicate that the brown algae known as bladderwrack, *Fucus vesiculosus,* is commonly used for producing kelp products.[4,5]

Kelp in the form of a powder or tablets is used in folk medicine to treat constipation, bronchitis, emphysema, asthma, indigestion, ulcers, colitis, gallstones, obesity, and disorders of the genitourinary and reproductive systems, both male and female. It is also claimed to "clean" the bloodstream, strengthen resistance to disease, overcome rheumatism and arthritis, act as a tranquilizer, combat stress, and alleviate skin diseases, burns, and insect bites.[4]

Many of these actions are attributed to kelp's content of minerals, especially iodine. But the concentration of iodine in seaweeds is extremely variable, not only among different species but within the same species. For example, we find *Fucus vesiculosus* grown in the Baltic Sea contained 0.03% iodine; that harvested from the North Sea yielded 0.1% and still other specimens up to 0.2%.[6] Other species of *Fucus* may contain as much as 0.5% iodine. Consequently, if a kelp preparation is to be taken for its iodine content, that should be standardized or at least determined and stated on the label.

One of the advocated uses of kelp is to control obesity. This role is attributed to the plant's iodine content which supposedly stimulates the production of iodine-containing thyroid hormones. However, such stimulation would only result in people suffering iodine deficiency, an almost unknown condition in this age of iodized salt. The required daily allowance of iodine in adults is quite small, not exceeding 150 micrograms; consequently, administering extra iodine beyond the ability of the thyroid to use it is essentially worthless. Even if it were effective, using increased amounts of thyroid hormones for weight reduction is not recommended.[7]

Claims are also made that iodine-containing kelp is useful as a blood-vessel cleanser in the treatment of atherosclerosis. Iodine therapy for atherosclerosis is currently controversial and cannot be recommended. When it is employed, precise doses which are not available in unstandardized kelp preparations are administered.

Many of the other medicinal uses of kelp are dependent on its content of algin (sodium alginate), a high molecular weight polysaccharide found in all brown algae in concentrations ranging from about 12 to 45%.[3] Algin forms viscous, colloidal solutions or gels in water and is the ingredient in kelp responsible for its bulk laxative and demulcent (soothing) effects.

Actions which cannot be explained on the basis of kelp's iodine or algin content are probably not substantial. It is frequently pointed out by advocates that potassium is present in kelp in relatively large amounts. While that is true, what is usually left unsaid is that the seaweed is also high in sodium (salt). Kelp should consequently be avoided by those who must restrict their salt intake. Aside from its modest utility as a bulk laxative and demulcent, kelp has no real therapeutic value and very little to recommend it. In addition, it tastes bad.

REFERENCES

1. Stedman's Medical Dictionary, 23rd Ed. Williams & Wilkins, Baltimore, 1976, p. 740.
2. Encyclopaedia Brittanica, Vol. 13. Encyclopaedia Brittanica, Chicago, 1952, p. 317.
3. V. J. Chapman: Seaweeds and Their Uses, 2nd Ed. Methuen & Co. Ltd., London, 1970.
4. G. J. Binding and A. Moyle: About Kelp, Thorsons Publishers Ltd., Wellingborough, England, 1974.
5. R. Lucas: Common and Uncommon Uses of Herbs for Healthful Living, Arco Publishing Company, New York, 1969, pp. 53–57.
6. P. H. List and L. Hörhammer, Eds.: Hagers Handbuch der Pharmazeutischen Praxis, 4th Ed., Vol. 4. Springer-Verlag, Berlin, 1973, pp. 1062–1065.
7. V. E. Tyler, L. R. Brady, and J. E. Robbers: Pharmacognosy, 8th Ed. Lea & Febiger, Philadelphia, 1981, p. 488.

LETTUCE OPIUM

This venerable fraud of a drug keeps coming back to confront us like the proverbial bad penny. Consisting of the dried milky juice or latex of several species of lettuce, it is collected from the stem of the plant which is cut off at the time of flowering. The source most commonly utilized is the so-called wild lettuce, *Lactuca virosa* L., but garden lettuce, *L. sativa* L., as well as the related species *L. serriola* L. and *L. altissima* Bieb., all members of the family Compositae, also yield the product. Lettuce opium is also known by the Latin title, lactucarium.[1]

Taken as a drug by the ancient Egyptians, lettuce opium was long thought to possess soporific (sleep-producing) properties; however, this was probably based on the similar appearance of the white milky juice exuded by the cut lettuce plant and that yielded by the opium poppy. The odor, taste, and general appearance of lactucarium also resemble those of opium.

Introduced into conventional American medicine in 1799 by J. R. Coxe, a Philadelphia physician, the use of lettuce opium as a sedative and pain-killer flourished for a century or so and then gradually lost favor. By the mid-20th century, the drug had fallen into obscurity. Then suddenly, in the mid-1970's it was resurrected as a legal psychotropic or mind-altering drug by members of the American Hippie Movement. Various lettuce opium preparations were widely advertised in counterculture publications, either as the pure material or combined with "potency enhancers" such as catnip and damiana. The products were intended to be smoked in order to produce a feeling of euphoria and well-being (a "high").[2] At the height of lettuce opium's popularity in 1977, one dealer was reported to be making $1500 profit *per day* from the sale of extracted lettuce products.[3]

Over the years, repeated attempts have been made to demonstrate sedative and pain-killing effects in lettuce opium and to identify active principles which might be responsible for them. As early as 1892, hyoscyamine was reported in extracts of various lettuce species but not in commercial lactucarium.[4] These observations have not been verified by subsequent investigations. An extensive pharmacological study of lettuce opium published in 1940 showed that the fresh milky juice contained two bitter principles, lactucin and lactucopicrin, which had definite depressant or sedative effects on the central nervous system in small animals.[5] However, these compounds were found to be quite unstable, and commercial lactucarium had little, if any, activity.

An evaluation of lettuce opium in 1944 caused Fulton to reach the following conclusion[6]: "Modern medicine considers its sleep-producing qualities a superstition, its therapeutic action doubtful or nil." More recently, Brown and Malone examined one of the modern lettuce opium preparations and concluded, "The analgesic, sedative and other attributes of lettuce opium lactucarium, seem to be based on fiction rather than fact."[7]

Although these conclusions are certainly factual, a rather startling revelation regarding the constituents of lettuce was made in 1981. Scientists reported that studies using an extremely sensitive radioimmunoassay technique detected minute amounts of morphine (2 to 10 nanograms per gram, dry weight) in both hay and *lettuce*.[8] However, before getting too excited over this discovery, remember that a nanogram is a billionth of a gram; also, similar small quantities of morphine were found in such unlikely natural sources as cow's milk and human milk. The amounts involved in either lettuce or milk would be far too small to exert any obvious physiological effect. Sensible people may continue to eat lettuce in their bacon and tomato sandwiches, but they will not smoke it in their pipes.

REFERENCES

1. M. Grieve: A Modern Herbal, Vol. 2. Dover Publications, New York, 1971, pp. 476–477.
2. B. Rosen: High Times No. 23: 84, 1977.
3. R. K. Siegel: In Drug Abuse & Alcoholism. S. Cohen, Ed., The Haworth Press, New York, 1981, p. 12.
4. T. S. Dymond: Journal of the Chemical Society, Transactions 61: 90–94, 1892.
5. A. W. Forst: Naunyn-Schmiedebergs Archiv für experimentelle Pathologie und Pharmakologie 195: 1–25, 1940.
6. C. C. Fulton: The Opium Poppy and Other Poppies, Bureau of Narcotics, U.S. Treasury Dept., U.S. Government Printing Office, Washington, D.C., 1944, pp. 62–63.
7. J. K. Brown and M. H. Malone: Pacific Information Service on Street Drugs 5(3–6): 36–38, 1977.
8. E. Hazum, J. J. Sabatka, K.-J. Chang, D. A. Brent, J. W. A. Findlay, and P. Cuatrecasas: Science 213: 1010–1012, 1981.

LICORICE

"Can we ever have too much of a good thing?"
Signor Licentiate Pero Perez
in *Don Quixote*

L icorice consists of the underground parts, technically the rhizome and roots, of varieties of *Glycyrrhiza glabra* L. (family Leguminosae) which possess a sweet yellow wood. It is often called licorice root or glycyrrhiza. The root has been used since very ancient times as a flavoring and for its expectorant and demulcent properties in the treatment of coughs and colds.[1]

A very confusing situation exists concerning much so-called licorice candy. A great deal of it contains little or no licorice whatsoever but derives its flavor from anise oil. The taste of licorice and anise do resemble one another, but in other respects, including potential toxicity, they are quite different. It is unfortunate that the more common, harmless anise flavor is almost always referred to as licorice.

Millions of pounds of licorice are imported into the United States annually, most of it originating in the eastern Mediterranean region. About 90% of it is used in flavoring tobacco products — cigarets, cigars, pipe tobaccos, and the like. The amounts used are very closely guarded trade secrets, but the noticeable sweetness and pleasant flavor of many commercial tobacco blends is due to licorice. It is also an ingredient in various pharmaceuticals, especially throat lozenges. Authentic licorice-flavored candy is far more popular in Europe, especially Britain, than in this country.

Much of the sweetness of licorice is due to glycyrrhizin, also known as glycyrrhizic acid, a saponin glycoside which occurs in the root in concentrations averaging between 5 and 9%. It is about 50 times sweeter than sugar and is available commercially in a form known as ammoniated glycyrrhizin.

During World War II, a Dutch physician noted that administration of licorice extract produced marked improvement in patients suffering from peptic ulcer, but serious side effects in the form of swelling of the face and limbs were also observed.[2] Since then, numerous reports of toxic effects have been recorded in the medical literature based on the observation of patients who ate large amounts of licorice candy over long periods of time. One man who had eaten two or three 36-gram licorice candy bars daily for six to seven years became so weak he could not get out of bed. He required hospitalization with intensive treatment for more than one month before recovering.[3] Another person, previously in excellent health, ate 700 grams (about 1.5 pounds) of licorice candy in a 9-day period. His condition necessitated four days of hospital treatment.[4] In a controlled experiment, about 100 to 200 grams of licorice twists (equivalent to 0.7 to 1.4 grams of glycyrrhizin) eaten daily for periods of one to four weeks produced serious symptoms in a group of volunteers.[5]

Another interesting case involved an elderly man who chewed eight to twelve 3-ounce bags of chewing tobacco daily and swallowed the saliva produced. He became so weak that he was unable to sit up or raise his arms above the horizontal position. There was prompt improvement when he was hospitalized and denied chewing tobacco. Tests revealed that the brand he had been consuming contained more than 8% of licorice paste and that his usage amounted to between 0.88 and 1.33 grams of glycyrrhizin per day, well within the toxic range.[6]

The medical literature refers to this condition as pseudoaldosteronism, meaning one similar to that brought about by excessive secretion of the adrenal cortex hormone, aldosterone. In the case of licorice, the syndrome is caused by glycyrrhizin, the structure and physiological effects of which are related to aldosterone or desoxycorticosterone. Symptoms resulting from excessive quantities include headache, lethargy, sodium and water retention, excessive excretion of potassium, high blood pressure, and even heart failure or cardiac arrest.[7]

One popular herbal cough remedy contains 1 ounce of licorice root in a quart of water. Directions suggest that one-half pint be drunk at bedtime with additional quantities as needed.[8] The half-pint dose could easily contain 0.5 gram of glycyrrhizin, and that daily amount might be doubled or tripled, depending on the frequency of use. At that rate of consumption, toxic effects could be observed after a single week. For persons suffering from high blood pressure or heart trouble, these could be serious.

Although licorice does have a flavor pleasing to many and may also have some utility in treating coughs as well as a number of other conditions,[9] it must be remembered that it is also a potent drug. Large doses over extended periods of time are quite toxic.

When it comes to licorice, the answer to Pero Perez's question is "Yes!"

REFERENCES

1. V. E. Tyler, L. R. Brady, and J. E. Robbers: Pharmacognosy, 8th Ed. Lea & Febiger, Philadelphia, 1981, pp. 68–70.
2. C. Nieman: Chemist and Druggist 177: 741–745, 1962.
3. J. W. Conn, D. R. Rovner, and E. L. Cohen: Journal of the American Medical Association 205: 492–496, 1968.
4. T. J. Chamberlain: Ibid. 213: 1343, 1970.
5. M. T. Epstein, E. A. Espiner, R. A. Donald, and H. Hughes: British Medical Journal 1: 488–490, 1977.
6. J. D. Blachley and J. P. Knochel: New England Journal of Medicine 302: 784–785, 1980.
7. Anon: Medical Letter on Drugs and Therapeutics 21(7): 30, 1979.
8. R. C. Wren and R. W. Wren: Potter's New Cyclopaedia of Botanical Drugs and Preparations, New Ed. Health Science Press, Hengiscote, England, 1975, p. 187.
9. R. F. Chandler: Canadian Pharmaceutical Journal 118: 420–424, 1985.

LIFE ROOT

All of the old-time beliefs about the medicinal properties of the plant Senecio aureus L. are so aptly summarized in two sentences contained in a turn-of-the-century "doctor" book that it is worthwhile to quote them here[1]:

Life-root exerts a peculiar influence upon the female reproductive organs, and for this reason has received the name of Female Regulator. It is very efficacious in promoting the menstrual flow, and is a valuable agent in the treatment of uterine diseases. A recent herbal, which provides much the same information, includes the statement[2]: "A most valuable herb indeed."

Life root, also known as golden senecio, ragwort, false valerian, and squaw weed is a perennial herb with bright yellow flower heads belonging to the family Compositae. It grows in swampy grounds and moist thickets throughout the eastern and central United States. Actually, the entire dried plant, not just the root, was used as a drug.[3] It is, for example, still one of the principal ingredients in that famous old proprietary remedy Lydia Pinkham's Vegetable Compound.[4]

Small but readily detectable quantities (0.006%) of the toxic alkaloid senecionine are now known to be present in life root.[5] Senecionine belongs to the group of hepatotoxic (poisonous to the liver) pyrrolizidine alkaloids which are effective in inducing chronic disease in rats with one, or at most, a few doses.[6] A strong possibility exists that such alkaloids are involved in human liver diseases, including primary liver cancer.

For this reason, it is not useful to discuss in detail the therapeutic potential of life root or the desirability of selfmedicating with it for conditions in which it may be effective. Because of the presence of senecionine, the drug is simply not safe to use. Its employment in herbal medicine should be discontinued as was its use, many years ago, in more conventional therapy.

REFERENCES

1. R. V. Pierce: The People's Common Sense Medical Adviser in Plain English: or, Medicine Simplified, 62nd Ed. World's Dispensary Printing Office and Binding, Buffalo, N.Y., 1895, pp. 341–342.
2. F. and V. Mitton: Mitton's Practical Modern Herbal, W. Foulsham & Co., London, 1976, p. 103.

3. H. W. Youngken: Textbook of Pharmacognosy, 6th Ed. The Blakiston Co., Philadelphia, 1948, pp. 889–891.
4. S. Stage: Female Complaints. W. W. Norton & Co., New York, 1979, p. 89.
5. R. H. F. Manske and H. L. Holmes: The Alkaloids, Vol. 1. Academic Press, New York, 1950, p. 159.
6. R. Schoental: In Chemical Carcinogens, C. E. Searle, Ed. American Chemical Soc., Washington, D.C., 1976, pp. 626–689.

LINDEN FLOWERS

A number of different species of the genus *Tilia* yield flowers which are used in folk medicine, but most of the commercial product is derived from *T. cordata* Mill. and *T. platyphyllos* Scop. Also known as basswood or lime trees, these are large deciduous trees of the family Tiliaceae which often grow over 100 feet. The former species is commonly referred to as the small-leaved European linden, the latter as the large-leaved linden. After collection in late spring, the yellowish or white fragrant flowers are rapidly dried in the shade. They must also be carefully preserved since even a small amount of moisture reduces their aromatic properties and their activity.[1]

Linden flower tea has been used since the late Middle Ages as a diaphoretic, that is, a drug which promotes perspiration. It is also recommended as both a nervine (tranquilizer) and a stimulant, two quite contradictory uses. In addition, it is considered valuable in the treatment of headaches, indigestion, hysteria, and diarrhea. Linden flowers were once thought to be so effective in the treatment of epilepsy that a patient could be cured simply by sitting under the tree![2]

A number of flavonoid compounds, particularly derivatives of quercetin and kaempferol, are found in linden flowers and, together with p-coumaric acid, are apparently responsible for the drug's diaphoretic properties. A pleasant-smelling volatile oil also occurs in the flowers along with quantities of tannin and mucilage.

Studies have shown that the relative amounts of tannin and mucilage are extremely important as far as the taste of linden flower tea is concerned. The taste becomes significant because relatively large amounts need to be drunk to induce perspiration. Flowers with a high tannin (2.0% or greater) and relatively low mucilage content produce a more tasty tea than those with a lower concentration of tannin and large amounts of mucilage. The latter tend to be quite insipid. This explains why the flowers of *T. cordata* and *T. platyphyllos* are preferred sources of the drug. They contain relatively more tannin and less mucilage than the flowers of such species as *T. tomentosa* Moench, the silver linden. Consequently teas prepared from the first two species taste much better.[3]

Authorities generally agree that linden flower tea is both a pleasant-tasting beverage and a useful diaphoretic.[4] The claims of therapeutic efficacy for other conditions should be disregarded. For the best-tasting product, select the flowers obtained from either *T. cordata* or *T. platyphyllos*. This may not be too easy if one has to rely on commercial sources which often fail to identify the botanical source. The flowers should also be stored in airtight, light-resistant containers in order to preserve their maximum fragrance.

There is no evidence to support the statement by Grieve that tea from very old linden flowers may produce symptoms of narcotic intoxication.[5] However, it has been reported that too-frequent use of linden flower tea may result in damage to the heart.[6] While this apparently occurs only occasionally and as a result of excessive intake of the beverage, those with known cardiac problems would do well to avoid using the drug.

REFERENCES

1. P. H. List and L. Hörhammer, Eds.: Hagers Handbuch der Pharmazeutischen Praxis, 4th Ed., Vol. 6C. Springer-Verlag, Berlin, 1979, pp. 180–184.
2. R. C. Wren and R. W. Wren: Potters New Cyclopaedia of Botanical Drugs and Preparations, New Ed. Health Science Press, Hengiscote, England, 1975, p. 184.
3. M. Luckner, O. Bessler, and P. Schröder: Pharmazeutische Zentralhalle 104: 641–644, 1965.
4. E. Steinegger and R. Hänsel: Lehrbuch der Pharmakognosie, 3rd Ed. Springer-Verlag, Berlin, 1972, p. 150.
5. M. Grieve: A Modern Herbal, Vol. 2. Dover Publications, New York, 1971, pp. 485–486.
6. M. Pahlow: Das grosse Buch der Heilpflanzen. Gräfe und Unzer GmbH, Munich, 1979, pp. 221–223.

LOBELIA

Throughout the 19th century, lobelia was such a favorite remedy of the practitioners of eclectic medicine that they were often called "lobelia doctors," a derogatory label. *Lobelia inflata* L. (family Lobeliaceae) with its erect branched stem, alternate ovate or oblong leaves, and small, pale blue flowers is quite an attractive plant. It is relatively common in the open woods and meadows of eastern North America but is also widely cultivated. The dried leaves and tops of the plant, also called Indian tobacco, make up the drug.[1]

Lobelia was valued primarily as a nauseant expectorant in cases of asthma and chronic bronchitis. In large doses, it acts as an emetic. Herbalists also report a beneficial action in conditions ranging from tuberculosis and nervous disorders to drug withdrawal,[2] but the drug's effectiveness in such cases is more imaginary than real. The renewed popularity of lobelia in recent years and its consequent inclusion in all the modern writings on herbs stems from its reputation as a euphoriant. Members of the counterculture smoke lobelia to obtain a mild, legal "high" analogous to that produced by smoking marihuana. The same feelings of mental clarity, happiness, and well-being are supposedly obtained by drinking lobelia tea or taking capsules of the powdered drug.[3]

The physiological activity of lobelia is accounted for by a mixture of pyridine-derived alkaloids contained in the plant to the extent of about 0.48%. Lobeline, lobelanine, and lobelanidine are the principal ones, with lobeline accounting for most of the drug's effects.[4] Less potent than nicotine but otherwise similar in its physiological action, lobeline first excites the central nervous system and then depresses it. In normal doses, it produces dilation of the bronchioles and increased respiration, but overdoses result in respiratory depression, as well as a host of other undesirable side effects including sweating, rapid heart beat, low blood pressure, and even coma followed by death. Large doses may cause convulsions.[5] Lobelia's value as an expectorant and treatment for asthma and bronchitis is limited by the tendency of the drug to upset the stomach. It is an effective emetic when administered in adequate quantity, but it is really not safe enough to use.[6]

Because of the similarity of its physiological effects to those of nicotine, lobeline is incorporated into tablets and lozenges usually containing 2 to 4 mg. of lobeline sulfate, which are claimed to help people stop smoking by masking the withdrawal symptoms of nicotine addiction. Unfortunately, the results of controlled trials with the drug have been disappointing.[4] Several of these proprietary products are nevertheless still marketed.

Self-administration in any form (smoking, drinking, eating) of inexact amounts of any crude drug as potent as lobelia is inadvisable. The ratio of risk to benefits is very high, especially when one considers the availability of much safer and effective treatments for any condition in which lobelia might conceivably prove helpful. Even the value of known quantities of lobeline as a smoking deterrent has not been proven. In short, the crude drug has been thoroughly discredited, and any use of it, either for therapeutic purposes or as a so-called euphoriant, is definitely not recommended.

REFERENCES

1. H. W. Felter and J. U. Lloyd: King's American Dispensatory, 18th Ed., Vol. 2. The Ohio Valley Co., Cincinnati, 1900, pp. 1199–1205.
2. L. Griffin: Herbalist 2(7): 4–7, 1977.
3. L. A. Young, L. G. Young, M. M. Klein, D. M. Klein, and D. Beyer: Recreational Drugs, Collier Books, New York, 1977, p. 114.
4. A. Y. Leung: Encyclopedia of Common Natural Ingredients Used in Food, Drugs, and Cosmetics, John Wiley & Sons, New York, 1980, pp. 225–226.
5. A. Wade, Ed.: Martindale: The Extra Pharmacopoeia, 27th Ed. The Pharmaceutical Press, London, 1977, p. 313.
6. T. Sollmann: A Manual of Pharmacology, 7th Ed. W. B. Saunders, Philadelphia, 1948, p. 352.

LOVAGE

A tall perennial herb with dark green leaves and greenish yellow flowers, *Levisticum officinale* W. D. J. Koch (family Umbelliferae) is extensively cultivated throughout much of Europe and the United States. In Europe, it is commonly known as the Maggi plant, sharing that name with the very popular, piquant flavoring sauce in which it is an important ingredient. All parts of the plant are highly aromatic with an odor and taste reminiscent of celery. The leaves are often used as a seasoning, especially for soups; the underground parts (rhizome and roots) constitute the drug.[1]

Since earliest times, particularly since the 14th century, lovage root has been a celebrated folk medicine, primarily for its diuretic and carminative properties. Besides increasing the flow of urine and expelling gas, it was thought to be of value for treating kidney stones, jaundice, malaria, sore throat, pleurisy, and boils.[2] Pahlow tells us that the root is still used in Europe for the self-treatment of stomach upsets, bladder and kidney problems, rheumatism, gout, menstrual disturbances, and migraine headaches.[3] Misled by the name lovage, many persons value the plant as an ingredient in love potions.

Lovage root contains 0.6 to 1.0% of a volatile oil, the principal constituents (70%) of which are a series of lactone derivatives known as phthalides. Some of the same constituents are also present in celery seed, thus explaining the similarities in taste and odor. Injection into rabbits and mice of small quantities of lovage extract and also of lovage volatile oil resulted in pronounced diuresis. Some dermatitis due to photosensitivity was also observed.[4] Sensitivity to light is a common phenomenon of umbelliferous plants as we have already mentioned with angelica. It apparently is not a serious problem, for lovage continues to be sold in Europe as the principal ingredient (some say the only active ingredient) in a lot of diuretic tea mixtures. Lovage is an important flavoring ingredient, too, in various liqueurs, herb bitters, and sauces.

The bulk of the evidence would indicate that lovage root does possess a definite diuretic action. It may also be helpful in relieving flatulence or gas. Agents which do this (carminatives), according to one of my old pharmacy professors, are drugs which "give the patient a good burp." There is no question that fresh lovage leaves or roots, chopped fine and cooked in various meat soups, stews, or the like, definitely enhance the flavor.

REFERENCES

1. E. Steinegger and R. Hänsel: Lehrbuch der Pharmacognosie, 3rd Ed. Springer-Verlag, Berlin, 1972, p. 427.
2. M. Grieve: A Modern Herbal, Vol. 2. Dover Publications, New York, 1971, pp. 499–500.
3. M. Pahlow: Das grosse Buch der Heilpflanzen. Gräfe und Unzer GmbH, Munich, 1979, pp. 219–221.
4. P. H. List and L. Hörhammer, Eds.: Hagers Handbuch der Pharmazeutischen Praxis, 4th Ed., Vol. 5. Springer-Verlag, Berlin, 1976, pp. 497–500.

MISTLETOE

The word "mistletoe" is about as nonspecific a term as you could possibly apply to a plant material. The addition of "American" or "European" helps a little. When properly used, American mistletoe refers to a single one of the more than 200 species of the genus *Phoradendron*. However, this species has three different scientific names, each of which is used more or less interchangeably. The most acceptable designation presently is *Phoradendron tomentosum* (DC.) Engelm. subspecies *macrophyllum* (Cockerell) Wiens, but this name is considered synonymous with *P. serotinum* (Raf.) M. C. Johnston and *P. flavescens* (Pursh) Nutt. At first glance, the nomenclature for European mistletoe seems simpler; it is *Viscum album* L.. But there are three subspecies commonly recognized: *album*, growing on broad-leaf trees; *abietis* (Wiesbaur) Abromeit, growing on silver fir; and *austriacum* (Wiesbaur) Vollmann, growing on various pines and spruces. All of the plants are parasitic shrubs belonging to the family Loranthaceae.

Although the berries of both American and European mistletoe have long been considered poisonous, the leaves, in the form of a tea, have a considerable reputation as a home remedy. The reputed uses of the two plants are as different as their names. American mistletoe is believed to stimulate smooth muscles, causing a rise in blood pressure and increased uterine and intestinal contractions. European mistletoe has precisely the opposite reputation of reducing blood pressure and acting as an antispasmodic and calmative agent.[1]

Actually, both kinds of mistletoe contain toxic proteins which are very similar in their chemical composition.[2] These are designated phoratoxin when isolated from *Phoradendron* species and viscotoxins when obtained from various subspecies of *Viscum album*. Contrary to the folkloric reputation of the respective plants containing them, phoratoxin and the viscotoxins produced similar effects when injected into test animals. These included hypotension, slowing and weakening of the heart beat, and constriction of the blood vessels in the skin and skeletal muscles.[3] However, it must be noted that the effects of these toxins following oral administration in human beings have not been studied.

Extracts of European mistletoe are sometimes employed in Germany in the treatment of malignant tumors. A sterile solution, available commercially, is injected either intravenously or into the tumor itself to provide palliative treatment for certain types of cancer.[4] The drug has not been approved for use in the United States. Such use of mistletoe extracts has led to identification in the plant of three lectins, that is, proteins which agglutinate red blood cells.[5] Many plant lectins are highly cytotoxic, and research is currently being conducted to determine their potential in cancer chemotherapy.

Certain Australian species of mistletoe have been shown to extract toxic principles, such as alkaloids and glycosides, from the host plants on which they grow as parasites. Thus mistletoes grown on *Duboisia* species contain toxic solanaceous alkaloids and those grown on oleander contain potent cardiac glycosides.[6] The identity of the host plants on which the parasitic mistletoe is found is therefore extremely important if the crude plant material is to be used as a medicine.

Many popular writers on herbs recommend mistletoe tea as a treatment for conditions from anxiety to cancer. Because of the relatively high price of coffee, some persons have even advocated it as a pleasant-tasting substitute. All of the recent scientific studies emphasize the similar toxic nature of plant material, especially the berries but also the leaves, from both American and European mistletoe. So the use of either product as a home remedy or as a beverage should definitely be avoided.

REFERENCES

1. P. S. Brown: Herbalist 1(12): 449–450, 1976.
2. S. T. Mellstrand and G. Samuelsson: European Journal of Biochemistry 32: 143–147, 1973.
3. S. Rosell and G. Samuelsson: Toxicon 4: 107, 1966.
4. H. Becker and G. Schwarz: Deutsche Apotheker-Zeitung 112: 1462–1465, 1972.
5. R. A. Locock: Canadian Pharmaceutical Journal 119: 124–127, 1986.
6. C. Boonsong and S. E. Wright: Australian Journal of Chemistry 14: 449–457, 1961.

MORMON TEA

Mormon tea is prepared from the fresh or dried stems of *Ephedra nevadensis* Wats., family Ephedraceae, a small erect shrub native to the desert regions of the southwestern United States and adjacent parts of Mexico. Called popotillo by the Mexicans, and Mormon tea, teamster's tea, or squaw tea by the early American settlers, it was once a very popular folk remedy for syphilis and especially, gonorrhea. Although its taste is quite astringent, those who become accustomed to it like it as a pleasantly refreshing beverage.[1] The name Mormon tea probably derives from its use as a caffeine-free thirstquencher.

Since 1552, the plant yielding Mormon tea has been recommended as being beneficial to health. Widely used by frontiersmen as a cure for venereal disease, it is also described as a remedy for colds and kidney disorders, and as a "spring tonic."[2] Spoerke attributes its activity to the presence of an undetermined amount of the alkaloid ephedrine, a drug which constricts the blood vessels, dilates the bronchioles, and stimulates the central nervous system.[3] Both Gottlieb[4] and Mowrey[5] state that Mormon tea's active constituent is not ephedrine but (+)-norpseudoephedrine, an even more potent central nervous system stimulant.

Actually, five different groups of investigators have been unable to detect the presence of ephedrine, (+)-norpseudoephedrine, or any other alkaloid in *E. nevadensis,* and we may safely conclude that the plant is alkaloid-free.[6] This is in keeping with all other North American species of *Ephedra* which are singularly devoid of alkaloids. Mormon tea does contain large amounts of tannin, in addition to a resin and a volatile oil.

Administration of a fluidextract and an infusion (tea) of the drug to human subjects produced definite, but relatively mild, diuresis. The tea, which contained more water-soluble principles, was more effective in this regard than the alcoholic extract. Some constipation, probably due to the tannin, was also noted. The investigators concluded that Mormon tea does not belong to the exceedingly active class of medicinal plants and that the properties usually attributed to it are already "well supplied by some well established therapeutic agent."[1]

This is sound comment. If you enjoy the astringent flavor of Mormon tea and are not concerned about its high tannin content, you will be satisfied. If you expect it to have any pronounced therapeutic effect, you will be disappointed.

REFERENCES

1. R. E. Terry: Journal of the American Pharmaceutical Association 16: 397–407, 1927.
2. W. H. Hylton, Ed.: The Rodale Herb Book. Rodale Press Book Div. Emmaus, Pa., 1976, pp. 513–514.
3. D. G. Spoerke, Jr.: Herbal Medications. Woodbridge Press Publishing Co., Santa Barbara, Calif., 1980, pp. 122–123.
4. A. Gottleib: Legal Highs, 20th Century Alchemist, Manhattan Beach, Calif., 1973, p. 37.
5. D. B. Mowrey: Herbalist 2(6): 26, 1977.
6. R. Hegnauer: Chemotaxonomie der Pflanzen, Vol. 1. Birkhäuser Verlag, Basel, 1962, pp. 460–462.

MUIRA PUAMA

Botanists have had almost as much trouble identifying the source of muira puama as zoologists have experienced in locating the Loch Ness monster. Although the existence of the plant (unlike that of the monster) is beyond dispute, it was once thought to derive from *Liriosma ovata* Miers or perhaps, *Acanthea virilis* (nomen nudum). Finally, scientists identified it as the stem-wood and root of two Brazilian shrubs, *Ptychopetalum olacoides* Benth. and *Ptychopetalum uncinatum* Anselmino. Both are members of the family Olacadeae.[1]

Also known as potency wood, the drug has a long history of use in Brazil as a powerful aphrodisiac and nerve stimulant. It is an ingredient in a number of proprietary remedies and folk medicines for sexual impotence. Muira puama is also touted for dyspepsia, menstrual irregularities, rheumatism, and paralysis caused by poliomyelitis, and as a general tonic and appetite stimulant.[2]

The drug is administered by mouth, either as a powder, an alcoholic extract, or a decoction (extract formed by boiling in water). An alternative method of obtaining the aphrodisiac effect is to bathe the genitals with a concentrated decoction. It is also applied locally to treat rheumatism and muscle paralysis.

Chemical studies show that muira puama contains as its principal constituent 0.4 to 0.5% of a mixture of esters, two-thirds of which is behenic acid, lupeol, and β-sitosterol; in the remaining portion, other fatty acids replace the behenic acid.[3] Other more-or-less routine plant constituents, such as volatile oil, resin, fat, tannin, various fatty acids, and the like have been isolated from muira puama.

None of the constituents in this drug is known to exhibit any pronounced physiological activity. This, plus the lack of any reported clinical testing of muira puama, causes us to view its reported effects with considerable skepticism. Until such tests have been carried out, no claims of efficacy or safety can be substantiated, and we must conclude at this point that potency wood is instead impotent.

REFERENCES

1. V. E. Tyler, L. R. Brady, and J. E. Robbers: Pharmacognosy, 8th Ed. Lea & Febiger, Philadelphia, 1981, pp. 491–492.
2. E. F. Steinmetz: Quarterly Journal of Crude Drug Research 11: 1787–1789, 1971.
3. H. Auterhoff and E. Pankow: Archiv der Pharmazie 301: 481–489, 1968.

MULLEIN

Verbascum thapsus L., the common mullein of the United States, is a wooly biennial herb belonging to the family Scrophulariaceae. During the first year, its large, hairy leaves form a low-lying rosette. In the spring of the second year, a tall stem develops from them to a height of 4 feet or more and is topped by a spike of yellow flowers. Both the leaves and flowers of this and of closely related Verbascum species have been used in folk medicine. The flowers are particularly popular in Europe and are usually obtained from V. phlomoides L. or V. thapsiforme Schrad., species native to that continent.[1]

According to Grieve,[2] mullein is valuable in the treatment of such a wide range of ailments as to make the newest "wonder drug" seem inactive in comparison. It is believed to possess demulcent, emollient, and astringent properties and is useful in treating both bleeding of the lungs (tuberculosis) and of the bowels. Not only is it both a sedative and a narcotic, but it can also be useful in treating cases of asthma, coughs, and hemorrhoids. Burns and erysipelas (streptococcus infections) yield to its application, as do bruises, frostbite, diarrhea, ear infections, most disease germs, and migraine. As if this were not enough — it is also useful in driving away evil spirits. This "wonder" drug is taken internally, applied locally, and even smoked, to treat these various conditions. Some of the more practical but less medicinal applications of mullein include using the yellow flowers as a blond hair dye and wearing the fuzzy leaves in the stockings to keep the feet warm.

Returning now to reality, a number of different chemical constituents, including a mucilage, saponins, and tannins have been identified in both mullein leaves and flowers.[3] None of these compounds in the quantities present possesses any important therapeutic activity, although they do have some mild demulcent (soothing), expectorant, and astringent properties. In Europe, the flowers are a common ingredient in many of the popular herbal mixtures sold as medicinal teas for their palliative effects in minor coughs and colds. In the United States, both the leaves and flowers formerly enjoyed official status in The National Formulary but were deleted in 1936, since except for its soothing mucilage, the drug lacked therapeutic virtue.[4]

REFERENCES

1. H. W. Youngken: Textbook of Pharmacognosy, 6th Ed. The Blakiston Co., Philadelphia, 1948, p. 800.
2. M. Grieve: A Modern Herbal, Vol. 2. Dover Publications, New York, 1971, pp. 562–566.
3. P. H. List and L. Hörhammer, Eds.: Hagers Handbuck der Pharmazeutischen Praxis, 4th Ed. Vol. 6C. Springer-Verlag, Berlin, 1979, pp. 417–422.
4. A. Osol and G. E. Farrar, Jr.: The Dispensatory of the United States of America, 24th Ed. J. B. Lippincott, Philadelphia, 1947, p. 1644.

MYRRH

. . . and looking up they saw a caravan of Ish-
maelites coming from Gilead, with their camels
bearing gum, balm, and myrrh, on their way to
carry it down to Egypt.

Genesis 37:25

Such quotations make us aware that myrrh has been an important article of commerce from ancient times; but it was valued then as a constituent of incense and perfumes, as well as one of the main ingredients in the embalming process, rather than as a medicinal agent. Technically, myrrh is an oleo-gum-resin (a mixture of volatile oil, gum, and resin) obtained from *Commiphora molmol* Engl., *C. abyssinica* (Berg) Engl. or other species of *Commiphora*. These are small trees of the family Burseraceae, native to Ethiopia, Somalia, and the Arabian peninsula. Myrrh consists of irregular masses or tear-shaped pieces, dark yellow or reddish brown in color, which exude naturally or from incisions made in the bark. The different commercial varieties are named according to their source, for example, Somali myrrh and Arabian myrrh.

Modern herbalists recommend myrrh as an antiseptic. It is incorporated into a salve which is applied externally in treating hemorrhoids, bed sores, and wounds. The tincture (alcoholic solution) is considered an effective oral astringent and is used as a mouthwash or for treating sore throat and similar conditions. Myrrh is taken internally for indigestion, ulcers, and to relieve bronchial congestion. It even enjoys some reputation as an emmenagogue (stimulates menstrual flow).[2,3] The suggestion that it can be therapeutic in cancer, leprosy, and syphilis is farfetched.[4]

Myrrh contains about 8% of a volatile oil, 25 to 40% of resin, and about 60% of gum. Various aldehydes and phenolic constituents in the volatile oil combine with acidic constituents in the resin to produce some astringent and antiseptic properties in the oleo-gum-resin. The physical properties of the gum and resin also confer a protective action on the mixture. Although myrrh is presently an ingredient in several commercial mouthwashes, it is far more widely used as a fragrance component in soaps, cosmetics, and perfumes and a flavor component in food products such as candy, baked goods, and so on.

Our ancestors, who valued the oleo-gum-resin primarily for its fragrance, were perhaps better informed about the appropriate use of myrrh than we are. As a drug, it is apparently relatively nontoxic but possesses only mild astringent and protective properties.

REFERENCES

1. V. E. Tyler, L. R. Brady, and J. E. Robbers: Pharmacognosy, 8th Ed. Lea & Febiger, Philadelphia, 1981, pp. 157–158.
2. M. Tierra: The Way of Herbs. United Press, Santa Cruz, Calif., 1980, pp. 105–106.
3. R. Lucas: Nature's Medicines. Wilshire Book Co., North Hollywood, Calif., 1977, pp. 71–75.
4. A. Y. Leung: Encyclopedia of Natural Ingredients Used in Food, Drugs, and Cosmetics. John Wiley & Sons, New York, 1980, pp. 241–242.

NETTLE

One would think that a high-technology society capable of splitting the atom and sending a man to the moon would long ago have learned everything there is to know about the stinging nettle. Not so. Even the agent responsible for the skin irritation produced by contact with the leaves of this common plant remains nearly as much a mystery to 20th century scientists as it did to the first cave man who stumbled against it. Its erect stalk, 2 to 3 feet in height, bears dark green leaves with serrated margins and small, inconspicuous flowers. Botanists now designate it Urtica dioica L. and place it in the family Urticaceae. (After accidental contact with it, people usually refer to the nettle by various uncomplimentary titles.)

The entire plant, collected just before flowering, has had a lengthy reputation in folk medicine as a specific for asthma. It has also been given as an expectorant, antispasmodic, diuretic, astringent, and tonic.[1] Applying nettle to the scalp, especially in the form of the fresh juice, is said to stimulate hair growth. Cases of chronic rheumatism have been treated by placing nettle leaves directly on the afflicted area. Roman soldiers, facing the inhospitable climate in Britain, reportedly used the same irritation produced by nettle leaves to keep their legs warm.[2] The tender tops of young first-growth nettles are believed especially palatable when cooked; Gibbons gives a number of recipes which utilize them, including nettle pudding and nettle beer.[3]

Numerous analyses of nettle have revealed the presence of more than 20 different chemical constituents[4]; none of them would provide any pronounced therapeutic activity from the plant when taken internally. Although the local irritation produced by the stinging hairs is real enough, there is just no evidence to show that it is effective in treating rheumatism or growing hair on bald heads. The principle(s) in the hairs thought to be responsible for this irritant action include histamine, acetylcholine, and 5-hydroxytryptamine. However, studies on plants of the closely related but more toxic genus Laportea have cast doubt on this, and the identity of the compound responsible for the pain from contact with nettle remains to be established.[5]

Many ancient and modern herbalists assert that rubbing fresh dock (Rumex) leaves on the affected area will reduce the stinging discomfort of nettle rash. There is even an old rhyme:

"Nettle in, dock out.
Dock rub nettle out!"

No objective evidence supports this claim aside from the fact that firm rubbing—by itself—was found to produce a short-lived lessening of the pain inflicted by *Laportea* species.[6] It is also possible that the time and effort spent on finding a dock leaf is sufficient to distract the victim from the itching caused by nettle rash.[7]

Nettle is rich in chlorophyll and serves as a readily available commercial source of that pigment. Young nettle shoots are edible when cooked and contain approximately the same amounts of carotene (provitamin A) and vitamin C as spinach or other similar greens. The diuretic properties of nettle have long been recognized, and several pharmaceutical preparations incorporating it are currently marketed in Europe for this purpose. Unfortunately, the folkloric claims of usefulness for a wide variety of other conditions require verification.

REFERENCES

1. M. Grieve: A Modern Herbal, Vol. 2. Dover Publications, New York 1971, pp. 574–579.
2. R. C. Wren and R. W. Wren: Potter's New Cyclopaedia of Botanical Drugs and Preparations, New Ed. Health Science Press, Hengiscote, England, 1975, pp. 216.
3. E. Gibbons: Stalking the Healthful Herbs, Field Guide Ed. David McKay Co., New York, 1970, pp. 133–138.
4. W. Holzner, Ed.: Das *Kritische* Heilpflanzen-Handbuch. Verlag ORAC, Vienna, 1985, p. 18.
5. W. V. MacFarlane: Economic Botany 17: 303–311, 1963.
6. W. V. MacFarlane: *In* Venomous and Poisonous Animals and Noxious Plants of the Pacific Region, H. L. Keegan and W. F. MacFarlane, Eds. Macmillan, New York, 1963, pp. 31–37.
7. J. Mitchell and A. Rook: Botanical Dermatology. Greengrass Ltd., Vancouver, B.C., Canada, 1979, p. 38.

NEW ZEALAND GREEN-LIPPED MUSSEL

An extract prepared from the New Zealand green-lipped mussel is the most recent "therapeutic substance" in a long line of such non-drugs advocated for the relief of symptoms of arthritis. The mussel, known technically as *Perna canaliculus*, a member of the family Mytilidae, is cultivated on special marine farms; at an unspecified time in its growth cycle, it is extracted by an undesignated process to yield a product of largely unknown composition which is stabilized by freeze-drying.[1] It is commonly marketed in the form of 250 mg. tablets.

Advocates maintain that daily doses of the extract relieve the discomfort of both rheumatoid and osteoarthritis in patients of any age without any dangerous side effects. They recommend taking the product for periods of 3 to 18 weeks and cite relief of pain, restoration of mobility and reduction of joint distortion, even in very elderly people who have been crippled for years with the disease. Mussel extract is also claimed to produce a feeling of well-being and a desire to be active. Sixty percent of persons treated are supposed to have shown improvement.

Croft indicates that how mussel extract works is unknown although he does note that it appears to work directly "on the origin of the inflammation rather than on the inflammation itself."[1] He further reports that although the extract contains amino acids and minerals, all attempts to fractionate it to obtain and identify an active principle have resulted in a total loss of activity. Long contradicts these statements, pointing out that the mussel extract contains mucopolysaccharides of the hyaluronic-acid type which act by increasing the viscosity of the joint lubricants in the body, thereby relieving swelling and stiffness. They also are believed to contribute to the extract's effectiveness in healing soft tissues, torn tendons, and bruises.[2] Yet there is no evidence to support the latter assertions. Although such mucopolysaccharides are important in forming the cement which binds body cells together and in producing other gel-like materials,[3] when taken by mouth they would be largely broken down by the digestive process prior to absorption and thus be unable to carry out these functions.

Scientific studies in small animals as well as clinical investigations in human beings have not produced any substantial evidence of the effectiveness of mussel extract for arthritis. No anti-inflammatory action could be demonstrated in rats when the extract was given to them orally. A 6-month clinical trial carried out on patients in a Scottish hospital seemed to have some positive results, but the "clinical data were poorly controlled."[4]

About the best that can be said for New Zealand green-lipped mussel extract for now is that, except in persons allergic to shellfish, it does not seem to have any pronounced toxicity nor to produce any serious side effects. It certainly has equally little in the way of therapeutic benefits.

REFERENCES

1. J. E. Croft: Relief from Arthritis: A Safe and Effective Treatment from the Ocean. Thorsons Publishers Limited, Wellingborough, England, 1979.
2. M. L. Long: Herbalist New Health, 6(4): 20, 1981.
3. C. H. Best and N. B. Taylor: The Physiological Basis of Medical Practice, 7th Ed. Williams & Wilkins, Baltimore, 1961, p. 21.
4. Anon.: Lancet 1: 85, 1981.

PANGAMIC ACID ("VITAMIN B$_{15}$")

> *"When I use a word," Humpty Dumpty said in a*
> *rather scornful tone, "it means just what I*
> *choose it to mean — neither more nor less."*
> Lewis Carroll
> *Through the Looking Glass*

Pangamic acid (variously known as vitamin B$_{15}$, pangamate, calcium pangamate, Russian formula, etc.) is one of those words referred to by Humpty Dumpty whose meaning varies according to its user's intent. As far as identity is concerned, it may mean almost anything; as far as therapeutic utility is concerned, it means absolutely nothing.

Originally, pangamic acid was the name given to a compound which Ernst Krebs, Sr. and Ernst Krebs, Jr. claimed to have isolated from the kernels of apricots (*Prunus armeniaca* L.) in 1943 and which was subsequently trade named by them as "vitamin B$_{15}$." Remember that Krebs, Jr. was the discoverer of laetrile, a product also obtained from apricot kernels. Pangamic acid was identified as *d*-gluconodimethyl aminoacetic acid, an ester of *d*-gluconic acid and dimethylglycine. A United States patent, issued in 1949, claimed that pangamate was able to detoxify toxic products formed in the human system. It was also supposed to be effective in treating asthma and allied diseases, conditions of the skin and the respiratory tract, painful nerve and joint afflictions, cell proliferation (cancer?), eczema, arthritis, neuritis, and the like. No scientific or clinical evidence was presented in support of these claims.[1]

At the present time, a number of companies market pangamic acid, but the true identity of the product is known only to Humpty Dumpty because it varies with the producer. Pangamic acid consists variously of one or more of the following ingredients, often simply mixed together: sodium gluconate, calcium gluconate, glycine, di-isopropylamine dichloroacetate, dimethylglycine, calcium chloride, dicalcium phosphate, stearic acid, Avicel (a form of cellulose), and so on.[2] Since there is absolutely no standard of chemical identity for products sold under the name pangamic acid (or any of its various synonyms), one authority takes the position that the preparation has no real existence.[1]

Unfortunately, the commercial tablets sold in various "health food" outlets under this name, and the exorbitant price charged for such products (about $10.00 for 100 tablets) are all too real. Besides, depending on its composition, pangamic acid may be toxic to human beings. Gluconic acid, glycine, and acetate are relatively inert, but isopropylamine acts on smooth muscle to lower blood pressure. Yet many of the advertisements for pangamic acid claim it improves oxygenation of the heart, brain, and other vital organs.[3]

Dichloroacetate may cause oxalic acid stones and other kidney problems; it has also been shown to be mutagenic by the Ames test and therefore has the potential to induce cancer. Dimethylglycine may react with nitrites in the intestine to form dimethylnitrosamine, a potent carcinogen. Calcium chloride also has poisonous properties.[1]

None of these constituents of the various pangamic acid products has been shown to have any nutritional or medical utility. Consequently, early in 1981, the FDA increased its seizures of the product after legal cases in several district courts had upheld the agency's actions in similar test cases. Unfortunately, the number of FDA seizures has been relatively small in comparison to the enormous amount of this totally worthless and potentially dangerous product offered for sale.[4,5] In 1987, pangamic acid was still being marketed throughout the United States, both as such and in the form of "equivalents," such as dimethylglycine.

REFERENCES

1. V. Herbert: Nutrition Cultism: Facts and Fiction. George F. Stickley Co., Philadelphia, 1980, pp. 107–120.
2. R. J. Moleski, Ed.: Informer (University of Rhode Island, College of Pharmacy, Drug Information Service) 3(6): 1–4, 1979.
3. J. B. Laudano: Recipe (St Johns University, College of Pharmacy and Allied Health Professions) 16(2): 7–8, 1979.
4. T. H. Jukes: Journal of the American Medical Association 242: 719–720, 1979.
5. Anon.: Drug Topics 125(5): 20, 1981.

PAPAYA

The papaya plant is a small tree, *Carica papaya* L. (family Caricaceae), native to tropical America but found in tropical areas throughout the world. Its trunk which is non-woody and hollow produces large, deeply lobed leaves and smooth-skinned cantaloupe-like fruits or melons directly on its surface without intervening branches. When ripe, the fruits are a very desirable food. Shallow cuts made on the surface of fully grown but unripe fruits cause them to exude a milky sap or latex which after collection and drying is known as crude papain. In addition to the large quantities produced by incising the fruit, about 2% of papain is found in papaya leaves.[1]

Papain, or vegetable pepsin as it is sometimes called, is a mixture of proteolytic enzymes with a fairly broad spectrum of activity; it hydrolyzes not only proteins but small peptides, amides, and some esters as well. Other components of the crude enzyme mixture hydrolyze both carbohydrates and fats.[2] This wide range of activity accounts for the use of papain in folk medicine for digestive disturbances of all kinds but particularly for those associated with protein-rich foods. The enzyme and the papaya leaves are also employed as a vermifuge (expels intestinal worms), especially for tapeworms.[3] As a digestive aid, papaya tablets containing between 10 and 50 mg. of papain are commercially available.

Face creams, lotions, cleansers, and so on are often formulated with papain in the belief that the enzyme will exert "a digestive effect on freckles and other sun blemishes" while cleansing the pores of make-up and providing a general "softening" effect. However, the use of papain most familiar to every housewife is as a *meat* tenderizer. The enzyme mixed with salt as an activator and a carbohydrate dispersing agent is sold in every supermarket. When shaken on tough meat before cooking, especially beef, it acts as an effective tenderizer by predigesting to some degree the fibrous animal protein. Various commercial applications of papain such as chillproofing beer and clarifying fruit juices are interesting but beyond the scope of this discussion.[1]

Those who drink a tea prepared from papaya leaves as a digestive aid should be aware that (according to French) the leaves should first have been subjected to a fermentation process similar to that used for black tea. This is said to facilitate extraction of the active principles by boiling water and to brew a much richer beverage than is obtained with ordinary dried papaya leaves.[1]

Unfortunately, papain is quite unstable in the presence of digestive juices, so its efficacy as a vermifuge or digestive aid is open to serious question.[4]

The 1978 report by Indian investigators that papain was teratogenic (produced birth defects) and embryotoxic (poisonous to the embryo) in rats needs verification before it can be given much credence. A more realistic concern is the enzyme's ability to induce allergic responses in sensitive individuals.[5]

REFERENCES

1. C. D. French: Papaya: The Melon of Health. Arco Publishing Co., New York, 1972.
2. V. E. Tyler, L. R. Brady, and J. E. Robbers: Pharmacognosy, 8th Ed. Lea & Febiger, Philadelphia, 1981, pp. 290–291.
3. M. Pahlow: Das grosse Buch der Heilpflanzen. Gräfe und Unzer GmbH, Munich, 1979, p. 405.
4. H. Wagner: Pharmazeutische Biologie: Drogen und ihre Inhaltsstoffe, 2nd Ed. Gustav Fischer Verlag, Stuttgart, 1982, pp. 306–307.
5. A. Y. Leung: Encyclopedia of Common Natural Ingredients Used in Food, Drugs, and Cosmetics. John Wiley & Sons, New York, 1980, pp. 255–257.

PARSLEY

Parsley is like the weather. Everyone knows about it, but no one does anything about it. Parsley is certainly our most familiar herb, widely employed as a culinary garnish for more than 2000 years, but it is seldom eaten.

The leaf, root, and fruit of *Petroselinum crispum* (Mill.) Nym. ex A. W. Hill (family Umbelliferae) have also been used for centuries in folk medicine. Botanists indicate that the plant's leaves are pinnate decompound, which simply means that they are divided and somewhat feather-like in their appearance. Since parsley can be identified by anyone who ever ate in a restaurant, here are the essentials: a widely cultivated, biennial herb with yellow flowers borne in clusters. Its fruits, commonly called seeds, are small, ovate, and grayish to grayish brown with alternating ribs and furrows.[1]

In classical medicine, parsley fruits were used primarily as a stomachic or carminative (aids digestion and expels gas), and the root as a diuretic (increases flow of urine). The plant also enjoyed some reputation as an emmenagogue and an abortifacient (stimulates menstrual flow and abortion).[2] While there may be some basis in fact for these uses of parsley, such attributes as a cure for diabetes, heart problems, liver ailments, and venereal disease are purely fanciful.[3]

Using parsley as a digestive aid, diuretic, and emmenagogue is based on its volatile oil content, the concentration of which varies from less than 0.1% in the root, to about 0.3% in the leaf, and from 2 to 7% in the fruit. As is the case with many plants which have been cultivated for centuries, many varieties of parsley exist. The chemical composition of the volatile oil obtained from some of these varieties is quite variable. So-called German parsley oil contains 60–80% of apiol (parsley camphor) as its principal component; French parsley oil contains less apiol but more (50–60%) myristicin, a compound originally found in nutmeg oil but very similar to apiol, both chemically and in its physiological action.[4] Both apiol and myristicin are uterine stimulants, accounting for the use of parsley volatile oil as an emmenagogue and for its misuse as an abortifacient.

Although it is not commonly eaten in quantity, parsley herb is a good natural source of carotene (provitamin A), vitamins B_1, B_2, and C, as well as iron and other minerals. It is therefore a good nutrient, especially when combined with bulgur and other ingredients in the tasty Middle East salad, tabbouleh — but as a drug, parsley is essentially worthless.

Because of their relatively high content of volatile oil, the fruits (seeds) may possess some stomachic and diuretic properties, but both such actions are relatively mild. Parsley volatile oil with its contained apiol and myristicin is toxic, and under no circumstances should it be administered to pregnant women.[5] So, while the parsley plant is of little medicinal value, its volatile oil is literally:

> "A remedy too strong for the disease."
> Sophocles
> Tereus, Fragment II. 589

REFERENCES

1. H. W. Youngken: Textbook of Pharmacognosy, 6th Ed. The Blakiston Co., Philadelphia, 1948, pp. 632–633.
2. V. E. Tyler, L. R. Brady, and J. E. Robbers: Pharmacognosy, 8th Ed. Lea & Febiger, Philadelphia, 1981, p. 492.
3. M. S. Keller: Mysterious Herbs & Roots. Peace Press, Culver City, Calif., 1978, pp. 264–279.
4. H. A. Hoppe: Drogenkunde, 8th Ed. Vol. 1. Walter de Gruyter, Berlin, 1975, pp. 817–818.
5. T. Sollmann: A Manual of Pharmacology, 7th Ed. W. B. Saunders, Philadelphia, 1948, p. 148.

PASSION FLOWER

T he passion flower derives its name from the imagined re-
semblance of its floral parts to the elements surrounding
the crucifixion of Christ. Its three styles represent the three
nails, its ovary looks like a hammer, the corona is the crown of
thorns, the ten petals represent the ten true apostles (excluding
Peter who denied Him and, of course, Judas), and so on. The
Moldenkes[1] remind us that the plant was unknown in biblical
times, and the fancied symbolism dates from 1610.

For many years, the dried flowering and fruiting top of the
perennial climbing vine *Passiflora incarnata* L. (family Passiflor-
aceae) has enjoyed a reputation as a calmative agent and sedative.
It was listed in *The National Formulary* from 1916 to 1936 but has
since fallen into disuse in this country. Without valid evidence to
support taking passion flower extract as a sedative or nighttime
sleep-aid,[2] the FDA has not recognized it as generally safe or
effective since 1978. Still, it continues to be incorporated into
quite a few sedative-hypnotic drug mixtures marketed in Europe.
A sedative chewing gum containing passiflora extract and vitamins was patented in 1978 in Romania.[3]

Constituents responsible for the pharmacological activity of
passion flower have been the subject of ongoing research
throughout most of this century. The plant does contain one or
more so-called harmala alkaloids, but their number and identity
are disputed. Besides, such alkaloids generally act as stimulants,
not depressants. A Polish report that both an alkaloid fraction and
a flavonoid pigment fraction produced sedative effects in mice
was subsequently followed up by Japanese investigators.[4] They
were able to isolate small amounts of the pyrone derivative maltol
from an alkaloid-containing extract of the plant. Maltol was
found to induce depression in mice and to exhibit other sedative
properties. The scientists concluded that the depressant effects of
maltol no doubt counteracted the stimulant action of the harmala
alkaloids but were not strong enough to explain the total sedative
effects of the plant extract. Further studies are obviously necessary before the active principles of passion flower can definitely
be identified.

Reports in the literature that passion flower contains toxic,
cyanogenic glycosides are misleading. Spoerke,[5] for example,
makes such a statement but has confused the medicinally used
passion flower, *Passiflora incarnata*, with the commonly culti-

vated, ornamental blue passion flower, *Passiflora caerulea* (*P. coerulea* L.). The latter species does contain cyanogenic glycosides, but the plant we have been discussing does not.[6]

Even though passion flower is not recognized as a safe or effective drug in the United States, it is an ingredient in many pharmaceutical products sold in Europe as sedatives.

REFERENCES

1. H. N. Moldenke and A. L. Moldenke: Plants of the Bible. Chronica Botanica Co., Waltham, Mass., 1952, p. xiv.
2. Federal Register 43(114): 25578, June 13, 1978.
3. F. Gagiu, T. Budiu, P. Lavu, and O. Bidiu: Romanian Patent No. 59,589, In Chemical Abstracts 89: 48897n, 1978.
4. N. Aoyagi, R. Kimura, and T. Murata: Chemical & Pharmaceutical Bulletin 22: 1008–1013, 1974.
5. D. G. Spoerke, Jr.: Herbal Medications, Woodbridge Press Publishing Co., Santa Barbara, Calif., 1980, pp. 134–135.
6. R. Hegnauer: Chemotaxonomie der Pflanzen, Vol. 5. Birkhäuser Verlag, Basel, 1969, p. 295.

PAU D'ARCO

Perhaps the most popular herbal cancer "cure" that has appeared in recent times is pau d'arco tea — also known as ipe roxo, lapacho, or taheebo tea. This beverage is prepared from the bark of various species of *Tabebuia*, a genus of about 100 broad-leaved, mostly evergreen trees of the family Bignoniaceae, native to the West Indies and Central and South America. Referred to in Brazil as ipe or pau d'arco, these plants have an extremely hard wood that is most attractive and practically indestructible.[1] Its resistance to decay probably attracted the attention of the natives to the medicinal potential of the species.

Popular reports state that Indian tribal doctors in Brazil brew a tea from the inner bark of *Tabebuia avellanedae* or *Tabebuia altissima*, known respectively as lapacho colorado and lapacho morado, which is used to treat cancer as well as ulcers, diabetes, and rheumatism. Proponents also claim that pau d'arco is "a powerful tonic and blood builder" and is effective against rheumatism, cystitis, prostatitis, bronchitis, gastritis, ulcers, liver ailments, asthma, gonorrhea, ringworm, and even hernias.[2,3] The drug is claimed to have been popular in the old Inca Empire, long before the Spanish invaded the New World. *T. avellanedae* is native to the warmer parts of the South America, but *T. altissima* supposedly grows high in the Andes Mountains where "not even the worst winter storms can blow it down."

Such popular reporting leaves much to be desired. There is no plant with the scientific name *Tabebuia altissima*; further, no species of *Tabebuia* grows high in the Andes. This remote habitat was apparently the creation of some advertising copywriter to make the drug sound more exotic. While *Tabebuia avellanedae* is a name found in literature, the correct botanical designation of the species is *Tabebuia impetiginosa* (Mart.) Standl.

Complicating the matter of origin even further is the fact that some of pau d'arco herbal teas marketed in this country do not derive from the *Tabebuia* species at all, even though they are labeled as lapacho colorado or lapacho morado. Instead, they are stated to represent the bark of *Tecoma curialis* Solhanha da Gama, another closely related member of the same plant family. This probably makes little difference because the useful constituents and therapeutic activities, if any, are undoubtedly similar. It nevertheless leaves the botanical source of pau d'arco products unclear. The outstanding American botanical authority on this group of plants, Dr. A. H. Gentry, speculates that probably all of the bark in question is being obtained from some lowland *Tabebuia* species.[4]

Because of their commercial significance in the construction industry, *Tabebuia* woods have been examined in detail. In addition to such therapeutically uninteresting constituents as volatile oils, resins, bitter principles, and the like, they contain from 2 to 7% of a napthoquinone derivative known as lapachol. Although few detailed studies of the chemical constituents of *Tabebuia* barks have been conducted, it is reasonable to assume that most of these barks contain lapachol as their principal active ingredient.[5]

Lapachol does possess some anticancer properties. In 1968 it was shown to have significant activity against Walker 256 carcinosarcoma, particularly when administered orally to animals in which this tumor had been implanted. In later studies, lapachol was found to be active against other kinds of animal cancers, including Yoshida sarcoma and Murphy-Sturm lymphosarcoma. In trials with human cancer patients, however, as soon as effective plasma levels were attained, undesirable side effects were severe enough to require that the drug be stopped. These included moderate to severe nausea, vomiting, anemia, and a tendency to bleed.[6] Animal and other laboratory studies have demonstrated that lapachol also possesses antibiotic, antimalarial, and antischistosomal properties, but scientific studies have not been done in humans because of the problem of toxicity.

Pau d'arco is marketed in the United States as a tea or "dietary supplement" with no therapeutic claims made on product labels. Its lack of proven effectiveness, its potential toxicity, and its relatively high cost render its use both unwise and extravagant.

REFERENCES

1. W. B. Mors and C. T. Rizzini: Useful Plants of Brazil. Holden-Day, Inc., San Francisco, 1966, p. 125.
2. A. de Montmorency: Spotlight January 5 and 12, 1981, pp. 10, 11, 34; June 8, 1981, p. 6.
3. B. Wead: Second Opinion: Lapacho and the Cancer Controversy. Rostrum Communications, Vancouver, B.C., 1985, 196 pp.
4. A. H. Gentry: Personal communication. September 9, 1983.
5. Anon.: Lawrence Review of Natural Products 4(9): 38–39, 1983.
6. J. B. Block, A. A. Serpick, W. Miller, and P. H. Wiernik: Cancer Chemotherapy Reports, Part 2 4(4): 27–28, 1974.

PENNYROYAL

Two very different members of the mint family (Labiatae) are referred to as pennyroyal. Although different in appearance, *Hedeoma pulegioides* (L.) Pers., the American pennyroyal, and *Mentha pulegium* L., European or Old World pennyroyal, possess similar chemical compositions and applications. A tea prepared from the leaves of either pennyroyal has been recommended as a stimulant, carminative, diaphoretic, and emmenagogue.[1] An emmenagogue promotes the menstrual flow but in popular writing is often a euphemism for an abortifacient. The more active pennyroyal oil has been taken in attempted abortion with tragic results.

American pennyroyal contains up to 2% of a volatile oil, and European pennyroyal up to 1% of an even more disagreeable-smelling volatile oil.[2] Both oils consist of 85 to 92% pulegone and are therefore quite toxic, causing severe liver damage even in relatively small amounts. Two tablespoonfuls of pennyroyal oil caused the death of an 18-year-old expectant mother in spite of intensive hospital treatment initiated just two hours after she took it.[3] As little as ½ teaspoonful of the oil has produced convulsions and coma in one individual.[4]

While pennyroyal oil may indeed induce abortion, it does so only in lethal or near-lethal doses. Such amounts would ordinarily not be obtained from drinking a tea prepared from the herb. Nevertheless, popular belief has it that pennyroyal tea is an effective abortifacient, as indicated by this description of the low upbringing of a virtueless woman:

> . . . she was the fifth of twelve children in the river-bottom family, with a mother who laid the cards and brewed tansy, pennyroyal, and like concoctions for luckless girls who were in need.

From *Slogum House* by Mari Sandoz*

Pennyroyal tea possesses no therapeutic properties which could not be obtained from more pleasant and effective medicaments. Therefore, the herb has little to recommend it.

---

*Copyright 1937, 1965 by Mari Sandoz. Published by the University of Nebraska Press. (By permission.)

REFERENCES

1. N. Coon: Using Plants for Healing, 2nd Ed. Rodale Press, Emmaus, Pa., 1979, p. 119.
2. E. Guenther: The Essential Oils, Vol. 3. D. Van Nostrand, New York, 1949, pp. 575–586.
3. J. B. Sullivan, Jr., B. H. Rumack, H. Thomas, Jr., R. G. Peterson, and P. Bryson: Journal of the American Medical Association 242: 2873–2874, 1979.
4. E. F. Early: Lancet 2: 580–581, 1961.

PEPPERMINT

B ecause it is such a popular flavoring agent and so widely used in just about every kind of product intended for human consumption, you would think peppermint was one of our oldest herbs. But it is not. The plant is a natural hybrid or cross which sprouted in a field of spearmint growing in England in 1696. Ever since that time, peppermint, Mentha piperita L. of the family Labiatae, has been intensively cultivated for its fragrant volatile oil. Since it does not breed true from seed, peppermint is vegetatively propagated; there are numerous cultivated varieties.[1]

Peppermint is used primarily for its stimulating, stomachic, and carminative properties in treating indigestion, flatulence (gas), and colic.[2] It is usually taken in a moderately warm tea prepared from the leaves, several cups being slowly sipped to bring fairly prompt relief. In Europe, the aromatic herb is incorporated in many tea mixtures intended to alleviate various ailments of the stomach, intestines, and liver. While it may well contribute to certain actions of these mixtures, it is often used simply as a pleasant flavor.

As an aid to digestion, its activity is due primarily to its contained volatile oil which exists in the herb (leaves and flowering tops) in concentrations ranging from 1 to 3%. American peppermint oil contains from 50% to 78% of free menthol and another 5% to 20% of various combined forms (esters) of menthol.[3] These major components are also largely responsible for peppermint's ability to stimulate the bile flow and promote digestion along with certain other flavonoid pigments with similar properties.

In addition, the volatile oil acts as a spasmolytic, reducing the tonus of the lower esophageal (cardial) sphincter and facilitating eructation (belching).[4] This antispasmodic property may also account for the popularity of peppermint tea as a household remedy for menstrual cramps. Peppermint oil temporarily inhibits hunger pangs in the stomach, but soon the stomach resumes its peristaltic movements which then become stronger than before.[5] In this way it works to stimulate the appetite.

Adults find peppermint tea to be a pleasant-tasting beverage and a useful remedy for mild digestive disturbances and related complaints. However, the tea should not be given to infants or very young children, since they may often experience a choking sensation from the contained menthol.

REFERENCES

1. M. Pahlow: Das grosse Buch der Heilpflanzen. Gräfe und Unzer GmbH, Munich, 1979, pp. 256–258.
2. M. Grieve: A Modern Herbal, Vol. 2. Dover Publications, New York, 1971, pp. 537–543.
3. V. E. Tyler, L. R. Brady, and J. E. Robbers: Pharmacognosy, 8th Ed. Lea & Febiger, Philadelphia, 1981, pp. 116–121.
4. P. H. List and L. Hörhammer, Eds.: Hagers Handbuch der Pharmazeutischen Praxis, 4th Ed., Vol. 5. Springer-Verlag, Berlin, 1976, pp. 767–771.
5. T. Sollmann: A Manual of Pharmacology, 7th Ed. W. B. Saunders, Philadelphia, 1948, p. 167.

POKEROOT

Pokeroot comes from *Phytolacca americana* L. (family Phyto-laccaceae), a large, much-branched, perennial herb which bears rather spectacular clusters of dark purple, almost black, berries. The plant is a wayside weed from New England to Texas. If there is any ailment for which pokeroot has not been recommended, it is simply because the herbalists have not yet thought of it. It is variously described as an alterative, cathartic, emetic, a narcotic, and a gargle, as well as a remedy for conjuncti-vitis, cancer, dyspepsia, glandular swelling, chronic rheumatism, ringworm, scabies, and ulcers.[1]

Pokeroot is not therapeutically useful for anything. It may act as an emetic and cathartic, but it does so because it is extremely toxic, due to the presence of a saponin mixture called phytolacca-toxin. The plant also contains a proteinaceous mitogen, PWM, which may produce various abnormalities of the blood cells after absorption.[2]

Children have died and adults have been hospitalized from the gastroenteritis, hypotension, and diminished respiration caused by eating pokeroot or the leaves of the plant. With the exception of the ripe berries, all parts of the mature plant are considered very poisonous. Some controversy exists about the relative toxicity of the berries, but they are nevertheless widely consumed as a folk remedy for rheumatism and arthritis. The very young shoots, which some use as potherbs, are believed to be innocuous. But it doesn't seem prudent to eat them when so many other safer sources of greens are available.

A 43-year-old Wisconsin woman recently drank one cup of tea prepared from a half teaspoonful of the root and required 24 hours of intense hospital treatment before her condition stabi-lized. As a result of this case, the Herb Trade Association issued a policy statement declaring that pokeroot should not be sold as an herbal food or beverage. It further recommended that all pack-ages containing it carry an appropriate warning statement re-garding the plant's toxicity and the potential danger if taken internally.[3]

With or without a warning label, pokeroot is definitely not recommended for either internal or external use by human beings. In the words of Lewis Carroll's Mad Gardener:

> 'Were I to swallow this,' he said,
> 'I should be very ill!'

REFERENCES

1. D. I. Macht: Journal of the American Pharmaceutical Association 26: 594–599, 1937.
2. W. H. Lewis and P. R. Smith: Journal of the American Medical Association 242: 2759–2760, 1979.
3. Anon.: Whole Foods 2(4): 14, 1979.

POLLEN

Exotic, even bizarre, remedies, ranging from peacock excrement to moss grown on the skull of a man who had died by violence, have long been part of our medical lore.[1] In fact, man has been extremely diligent in searching out such unusual materials, possibly in the hope that they may possess unusual curative properties. Pollen is a relatively recent example of such a drug. Although pollen extracts have been used for many years to detect and provide immunity against allergies, it is only during the past few years that pollen itself has become widely available in the form of tablets, capsules, extracts, and the like, which are recommended for a variety of ailments.

Pollen consists of microspores (male reproductive elements) of seed-bearing plants. Often the marketed product is designated bee pollen, implying that a mixture of pollens from various plants was collected by honeybees. Indeed, a mesh-like pollen trap has been developed which relieves bees of a portion of the pollen carried on their back legs as they reenter the hive. But there is no way to determine if a particular pollen grain was originally collected by a bee or not, so it seems best to refer to the commercially available material simply as pollen.

Enthusiasts declare that pollen will either provide relief for or cure such conditions as premature aging, cerebral hemorrhage, bodily weakness, anemia, weight loss, enteritis, colitis, and constipation.[2] It is also touted as having general tonic properties — promoting better health along with happiness and optimism. Studies conducted in Sweden and Japan seem to indicate the drug may be of value in treating chronic prostatism. An Austrian report found pollen useful in alleviating the symptoms of radiation sickness in patients being treated for cancer of the cervix.[3]

The chemical constituents of pollen have been rather extensively investigated. Although the different components vary greatly in quantity among pollens of different species, some general ranges may be quoted. Polysaccharides, particularly starch and cell-wall constituents, constitute up to 50% of a typical pollen. Low-molecular-weight carbohydrates (simple sugars) make up another 4–10%. The concentration of lipids (fats, oils, and waxes) is extremely variable, ranging from 1–20%. Protein exists to the extent of 5.9–28.3%, but only 0.5–1.0% of the total protein is allergenic in nature. About 6% of free amino acids are also present. Other constituents include about 0.2% of carotenoid and flavonoid pigments plus small amounts of terpenes and sterols. Some pollens are quite high in vitamin C; concentrations ranging from 3.6–5.9% have been reported.[4]

None of the identified constituents of pollen has been linked to any significant therapeutic activity as advocated by its enthusiasts. The few studies where favorable results were obtained require repetition and reevaluation before being accepted as factual. In the meantime, keep in mind that many pollens can induce severe allergic responses when inhaled or eaten, at least in some individuals.

Pollen's continuing appeal to an uncritical public was demonstrated recently when a snack bar containing it was chosen as the "official snack food" of the 1987 Pan American Games in Indianapolis. After the bee pollen in the bars was found to contain ragweed pollen, a serious, perennial allergen for many Indiana residents, the product was widely denounced by nutritionists and FDA officials. The producer claimed the bars provided an "energy boost" lasting for several hours; authorities noted that this effect was due to the honey and other carbohydrates, not to the small amount of pollen, contained in the snack.[5]

Since pollen has no significant therapeutic or nutritive value which cannot be obtained more easily and cheaply from other sources, it cannot be recommended for either purpose. And since its allergenic properties may render it downright hazardous to some, we must actively discourage its use both as a medicine and as a food.

REFERENCES

1. A. C. Wootton: Chronicles of Pharmacy, Reprint Ed., Vol. 2. USV Pharmaceutical Corp., Tuckahoe, N.Y., 1972, pp. 2–3.
2. G. J. Binding: About Pollen. Thorsons Publishers Ltd., Wellingborough, England, 1971.
3. Anon.: Bee Pollen — A Short Treatise. Les Ruchers de la Côte d'Azur, New York, 1977.
4. R. G. Stanley and H. F. Linskens: Pollen. Springer-Verlag, New York, 1974.
5. L. G. Caleca: The Indianapolis Star, December 8, 1986, pp. 15–16.

PROPOLIS

Unlike pollen, of relatively recent medicinal use, propolis or bee glue was an official drug in the London pharmacopeias of the 17th century.[1] However, there was a long hiatus in its popularity between the 17th and the late 20th century; now propolis once again is receiving considerable attention from laymen and scientists both. The unusual drug is a brownish resinous material collected by bees from the buds of various poplar and conifer trees and used by the insects to fill cracks or gaps in their hives.

Those who advocate its therapeutic use claim that propolis has an antibacterial activity greater than that of penicillin and other common antibiotic drugs.[2] They maintain the product "works" by raising the body's natural resistance to infection through stimulation of the immunity system. It is supposed to be especially beneficial in the treatment of tuberculosis. Duodenal ulcers and gastric disturbances are also thought to benefit from propolis therapy. Applied externally in the form of a cream, advocates say it relieves various types of dermatitis, especially those caused by bacteria and fungi.[3] Propolis is commercially available in the form of capsules (both pure and combined with 50% pollen), throat lozenges, cream, chips (used like chewing gum), and as a powder (to prepare a tincture).

More than 25 different constituents of propolis have now been tested scientifically against various species of bacteria and fungi for antibacterial and antifungal effects. Results indicate that the antimicrobiual properties of the drug are attributable mainly to the flavonoids pinocembrin, galangin, pinobanksin, and pinobanksin-3-acetate; in addition p-coumaric acid benzyl ester and a caffeic acid ester mixture were also active. Pinocembrin, a 5,7-dihydroxyflavanone, showed considerable antifungal activity. However, none of these isolated principles was as effective as various antibiotics or sulfa drugs with which they were compared: streptomycin, oxytetracycline, chloramphenicol, nystatin, griseofulvin, and sulfamerazine.[4] A series of studies on propolis carried out in recent years by Polish investigators showed that besides bacteriostatic and fungistatic properties, the drug inhibited the growth of protozoa, accelerated bone formation, had regenerative effects on tissues, stimulated some enzyme actions, and showed cytostatic effects (inhibited cell growth and division).[5] It must be emphasized that all of these results were obtained from experiments carried out *in vitro*, that is, in the chemical laboratory outside the living body, or in small animals. Double-blind clinical trials in human beings have apparently never been conducted with propolis.

The flavonoid pigments of propolis seem to possess modest antibacterial and antifungal properties but much less active than the standard drugs for controlling such microorganisms. Other tentative claims for potential therapeutic utility require clinical verification. In the interim, it is safe — and appropriate — to continue using propolis to seal openings in bee hives, where it has proven highly effective.

REFERENCES

1. A. C. Wootton: Chronicles of Pharmacy, Reprint Ed. Vol. 2. USV Pharmaceutical Corp., Tuckahoe, N.Y., 1972, p. 2.
2. S. S. Jones: Whole Foods 3(9): 26–30, 1980.
3. T. Smith and S. S. Jones: Herbalist 4(11): 12–13, 1979.
4. J. Metzner, H. Bekemeier, M. Paintz, and E. Schneidewind: Die Pharmazie 34: 97–102, 1979.
5. B. Hladoń, W. Bylka, M. Ellnain-Wojtaszek, L. Skrzypczak, P. Szafarek, A. Chodera, and Z. Kowalewski: Arzneimittel-Forschung 30: 1847–1848, 1980.

RASPBERRY

Although the flavorful fruits of the red raspberry, varieties of *Rubus idaeus* L. (family Rosaceae), were once used rather extensively to give a pleasant taste to various pharmaceutical preparations, it is the leaves of the plant which are still used as a popular folk remedy. This prickly stemmed shrub, so familiar to many berry pickers, is a native of Europe but is now cultivated throughout the world.

Raspberry leaves are employed for their astringent and stimulant properties.[1] Supporters recommend a strong infusion (tea) as a gargle or mouthwash for sore mouth and inflammation of the mucous membrane of the throat as well as for various wounds and ulcers when applied locally to them. The moistened leaves may also be applied externally as a poultice. Drinking cold raspberry leaf tea as a remedy for diarrhea is said to give immediate relief to that and to various stomach ailments.

Incidentally, with one exception, the leaves of blackberry (*Rubus fruticosus* L.) are used in a similar fashion to raspberry leaves.[2] All of the comments about raspberry's astringent properties apply to both drugs. With respect to raspberry leaves, however, it must be noted that tea made from them has acquired a considerable reputation as "the drink" for expectant mothers. In the popular literature the beverage is praised as a "panacea during pregnancy which is said to do everything for allaying morning sickness to preventing miscarriage to erasing labor pains."[3] Even a reputable scientific reference credits it as a traditional remedy for painful and profuse menstruation and for use before and during confinement.[4]

The raspberry leaves' astringent properties for treating sore mouth or diarrhea, etc., are readily explained by an appreciable content of hydrolyzable tannin, containing both gallic and ellagic acids in the free and combined forms.[5] Without adequate clinical studies, it is impossible to say if the drug's reputation as a relaxant of the smooth muscles of the uterus and intestine is real or imagined. In any event, no chemical constituent of raspberry leaves capable of inducing such activity has ever been identified. Like most green leafy plant materials, fresh raspberry leaves contain quantities of vitamin C. How much is present in the commercially available dried leaves depends on the conditions of drying and the manner and time of storage.

At present, we lack sufficient evidence to support any real

therapeutic importance of raspberry. It does have an astringent action and might be called upon occasionally as a modestly effective mouthwash and gargle or diarrhea treatment. If pregnant women believe that it provides relief from various unpleasant effects associated with their condition, no harm is done because it is relatively inexpensive and, as far as we now know, relatively harmless except for its tannin content.

Incidentally, if you wish to purchase raspberry tea for its supposedly beneficial effects, be sure to read the label carefully and make certain that raspberry leaves are the principal ingredient. Many so-called raspberry teas are simply ordinary black teas flavored with a volatile oil that smells like raspberry fruits. Raspberry leaves do not have this characteristic fruity aroma. In my personal opinion, the best thing about raspberry is its fresh fruit, which I still like on my breakfast cereal.

REFERENCES

1. M. Grieve: A Modern Herbal, Vol. 2. Dover Publications, New York, 1971, pp. 671–672.
2. M. Pahlow: Das grosse Buch der Heilpflanzen. Gräfe und Unzer GmbH, Munich, 1979, pp. 164–166.
3. T. Clifford: Cures. Macmillan Publishing Co., Inc., New York, 1980, p. 52.
4. J. E. F. Reynolds, Ed.: Martindale: The Extra Pharmacopoeia. 28th Ed. The Pharmaceutical Press, London, 1982, p. 1751.
5. P.H. List and L. Hörhammer, Eds.: Hagers Handbuch der Pharmazeutischen Praxis, 4th Ed., Vol. 6B. Springer-Verlag, Berlin, 1979, 186–188.

RED BUSH TEA

It is a pleasure, for a change, to discuss a plant material which has no therapeutic value and for which none is claimed. Indeed, red bush or rooibos tea is valued not only for its taste but also because it is devoid of any undesirable physiological effects. Although there has been much confusion about the proper name of the plant whose dried leaves and fine twigs constitute the tea, it is now generally agreed to be *Aspalathus linearis* (Burm. f.) R. Dahlgr., also sometimes designated *Borbonia pinifolia* Marloth or *Aspalathus contaminata* (Thunb.) Druce.[1]

This member of the family Leguminosae is a shrub, native to the mountainous regions of South Africa. It attains a height of six feet and bears long needle-like leaves that turn a brick red color when bruised. The plant is now extensively cultivated, particularly in the Cedarberg Mountains near the Clanwilliam district. In late summer or early autumn, the plants are harvested, cut into short lengths, moistened, bruised, allowed to ferment, and dried in the sun to produce red bush tea which is brewed like ordinary tea to make South Africa's most popular hot beverage.[2]

Red bush tea is drunk either plain or with sugar and milk according to the consumer's taste. It is valued highly not only for its refreshing flavor—a liking for it may be acquired—but because it is low in tannin (less than 5%) and is essentially caffeine-free. These factors combine with the presence of some vitamin C in the tea (0.0016%) to produce a beverage which is quite acceptable to those who wish to avoid caffeine and high tannin concentrations in their hot drinks. Red bush tea is currently marketed in the United States under the trade name Kaffree® Tea.

REFERENCES

1. R. Dahlgren: Botaniska Notiser 117: 188–196, 1964.
2. R. H. Cheney and E. Scholtz: Economic Botany 17: 186–194, 1963.

RED CLOVER

During the early years of the 20th century, more than a half-dozen major pharmaceutical companies manufactured and marketed various "Trifolium Compound" preparations. The formula of one extract produced by the Wm. S. Merrell Chemical Co. of Cincinnati included red clover, the blossoms of *Triofolium pratense* L., plus seven other vegetable drugs. This extract and the fluidextracts and syrups of other manufacturers were widely sold as alternatives, that is, cures for venereal disease.[1] As early as 1912, the Council on Pharmacy and Chemistry of the American Medical Association reported,[2] "We have no information to indicate that they [red clover preparations] possess medicinal properties." Still, trifolium continued to be listed in *The National Formulary* until 1946.

A 1981 catalog of "health products" lists Red Clover Combination tea in which red clover is combined with four of the seven herbs contained in the previously discredited mixture, plus a few additional ingredients, added primarily for flavor.[3] As is customary in such publications, no therapeutic use is described, but the $16.00 price tag indicates the product should be good for something. Reference to a typical modern herbal will of course reveal that red clover is an alterative.[4] All this is reminiscent of the expression (attributed to Marie Antoinette's milliner), "There is nothing new except what is forgotten." Unfortunately, in this case, what had been forgotten should have remained forgotten.

The characteristic red blossoms of this extensively cultivated forage plant have been subjected to detailed chemical analyses. More than one-third of a page of fine print in a recent reference is required just to list the names of the chemical compounds detected in red clover.[5] Yet none of these various pigments, phenolic compounds, tannins and the like, has any pronounced therapeutic value, particularly in the treatment of venereal disease.

The statement that red clover tea sweetened with honey and drunk two or three times a day for a period of four to six weeks will purify the blood (euphemism for cure venereal disease) is simply not factual.[6] It is true that the obvious symptoms of the disease may disappear in that time, but no cure has been obtained.

This emphasizes one of the real dangers of self-medicating with ineffectual drugs. They themselves may not be harmful, but neglecting effective treatment for a serious disease may eventually prove disastrous. Exactly the same precaution applies to the local application of red clover flowers to treat "cancerous growths."[4] The herb is *not* effective in such conditions, and delay in obtaining proper therapy may be fatal.

REFERENCES

1. H. W. Felter and J. U. Lloyd: King's American Dispensatory, 18th Ed., Vol. 2. The Ohio Valley Co., Cincinnati, 1900, pp. 1995–1996,
2. A Reprint of the Reports of the Council on Pharmacy and Chemistry of the American Medical Association with the Comments that Appeared in the Journal During 1912, American Medical Association, Chicago, 1913, p. 40.
3. Swanson Health Products, Fargo, N.D., 1981, p. 18.
4. M. Grieve: A Modern Herbal, Vol. 1. Dover Publications, New York, 1971, pp. 207–208.
5. P. H. List and L. Hörhammer, Eds.: Hagers Handbuch der Pharmazeutischen Praxis, 4th Ed., Vol. 6C. Springer-Verlag, Berlin, 1979, pp. 265–266.
6. M. Pahlow: Das grosse Buch der Heilpflanzen. Gräfe und Unzer GmbH, Munich, 1979, pp. 352–353.

ROSE HIPS

Because of their relatively high content of vitamin C, the bright scarlet to deep red, ovoid or pear-shaped fruits or hips of several species of roses always occupy a significant place in discussions of natural medicines. Most commonly, the hips are collected from the dog rose *Rosa canina* L., but the larger hips of the Japanese rose, *R. rugosa* Thunb., are valued highly, as are those of *R. acicularis* Lindl. and *R. cinnamomea* L. All are more or less familiar members of the family Rosaceae.[1]

Rose hips are used to prepare teas, extracts, purees, marmalades, even soups, all of which are consumed for their vitamin C content.[2] The extracts are also incorporated into a number of "natural" vitamin preparations, including tablets, capsules, syrups, and the like. Most such preparations are careful not to state on the label exactly how much of the vitamin C content is derived from rose hips and how much from synthetic ascorbic acid. In addition to their antiscorbutic (antiscurvy) properties, rose hips have a mild laxative and slight diuretic action.

Although fresh rose hips contain concentrations of vitamin C ranging from 0.5 to 1.7%, the actual content of the commercially available dried fruit is extremely variable depending on the exact botanic source, where it was grown, when it was collected, how it was dried, and when and where it was stored, etc. Indeed, many commercial samples of the plant material no longer contain detectable amounts of vitamin C. Even if we assume that they contain an average of 1% of the vitamin and that all of the vitamin is present in the finished preparation—two propositions that are not necessarily valid—the present cost of vitamin C from rose hips is about 25 times more than the synthetic product.[3]

Rose hips contain, in addition to vitamin C, a large number of different chemical compounds including about 11% of pectin and 3% of a mixture of malic and citric acids. These are probably responsible for the mild laxative and diuretic effects of the drug.[4]

Based solely on cost, one must reject rose hips as an economical source of vitamin C. Of course, if you are able to collect and process your own, or if you simply like the taste of rose hips tea or similar preparations, that's quite a different matter. If you are still interested in the commercial product for its vitamin content—in spite of the cost—I would not recommend purchase unless the material is clearly labeled as to the amount of natural vitamin C actually contained in it. This is really asking very little. Relatively simple assay procedures exist,[4] and any well-equipped food or drug quality-control laboratory is capable of conducting them. Only in this way can you be assured of value received for any money you spend on rose hips.

REFERENCES

1. N. Coon: Using Plants for Healing, 2nd Ed. Rodale Press, Emmaus, Pa., 1979, p. 174.
2. J. C. Torke: Herbalist 1: 472–473, 1976.
3. V. E. Tyler, L. R. Brady, and J. E. Robbers: Pharmacognosy, 8th Ed. Lea & Febiger, Philadelphia, 1981, p. 494.
4. P. H. List and L. Hörhammer, Eds.: Hagers Handbuch der Pharmazeutischen Praxis, 4th Ed., Vol. 6B. Springer-Verlag, Berlin, 1979, pp. 164–170.

ROSEMARY

While it may be useful in the culinary art, rosemary is not one of the most valuable herbs from the medicinal viewpoint. That it is one of the best known is attested to by frequent references, some occurring even in children's literature.

> Old Mrs. Rabbit was a widow; she earned her living by knitting. . . . She also sold herbs, and rosemary tea . . .
> Beatrix Potter
> *The Tale of Benjamin Bunny*

Rosemary consists of the leaves or the leaves with flowering tops of *Rosmarinus officinalis* L. (family Labiatae), an evergreen shrubby herb with aromatic linear leaves, which are dark green above and white below, and small pale-blue flowers. It has been extensively cultivated in so-called kitchen gardens. If members of the women's liberation movement were to seek a plant to represent their cause, it would certainly be rosemary, for there is an old English belief that the plant will thrive only in the garden of a household where the "mistress" is really the "master."[1]

Various preparations of rosemary, including an infusion or tea, a wine, a spirit (alcoholic solution), and a bath, are recommended for their tonic, astringent, and diaphoretic (increases perspiration) effects. The leaves are also said to have stomachic (aids digestion) properties and to make a hair tonic which, when applied externally, will prevent baldness.[2] Rosemary is recommended especially in cases of low blood pressure; a bath prepared from it is so stimulating to the body that it should not be taken in the evening or it may prevent one from sleeping.[3] Finally, both the drug and its volatile oil have been used as emmenagogues (to stimulate menstrual flow) and abortifacients.

Whatever physiological activity rosemary possesses is attributed to its volatile oil which occurs in the leaves in concentrations ranging from 1 to 2.5%.[4] Containing such compounds as camphor, borneol, and cineole, the volatile oil, like many others, has antibacterial properties. It also has some stimulating properties, particularly when applied locally. The leaves of rosemary contain a number of flavonoid pigments, one of which, diosmin, is reported to decrease capillary permeability and fragility.[5] However, the exact extent of rosemary's therapeutic usefulness remains unknown, for no clinical studies with the leaves have been reported.

Rosemary is extensively used as a household spice and as a flavoring agent in various commercial products including prepared meats, baked goods, vegetables, and so on. It is far more useful for these purposes than as a medicine. Rosemary oil is widely employed as a fragrance component in soaps, creams, lotions, perfumes, and toilet waters; small amounts are also added as a flavoring agent to alcoholic beverages, frozen desserts, candy, puddings, and similar products. However, the larger quantities of the oil necessary for therapeutic purposes are not safe when taken internally and produce irritation of the stomach, intestines, and kidneys.[3] Besides, using rosemary as an abortifacient is certainly not a valid usage. Just what was old Mrs. Rabbit doing, selling that rosemary tea?

REFERENCES

1. M. Grieve: A Modern Herbal, Vol. 2. Dover Publications, New York, 1971, pp. 681–683.
2. R. C. Wren and R. W. Wren: Potter's New Cyclopaedia of Botanical Drugs and Preparations, New Ed. Health Science Press, Hengiscote, England, 1975, p. 261.
3. M. Pahlow: Das grosse Buch der Heilpflanzen. Gräfe und Unzer GmbH, Munich, 1979, pp. 270–272.
4. P. H. List and L. Hörhammer, Eds.: Hagers Handbuch der Pharmazeutischen Praxis, 4th Ed., Vol. 6B. Springer-Verlag, Berlin, 1979, pp. 172–176.
5. A. Y. Leung: Encyclopedia of Common Natural Ingredients Used in Food, Drugs, and Cosmetics, John Wiley & Sons, New York, 1980, pp. 283–285.

ROYAL JELLY

The newspaper headline read "Battling Budapest Baldies Briskly Buy Banfi," and the story which followed told how Hungarian men were engaging in brawls and fistfights to get a place in line so they might spend the equivalent of $2.85 to buy a bottle of the latest herbal hair restorer—a bottle which might be sold on the blackmarket for as much as $100. The exact formula of the "wonder" remedy concocted by promoter Andras Banfi was a secret, of course, but those in the know speculated that it contained egg yolk, orange tincture, alcohol, and royal jelly.[1]

Royal jelly is a milky white, viscous secretion produced by the pharyngeal glands of the worker bee, *Apis mellifera* L., an insect belonging to the family Apidae. During the first three days of life, all bee larvae feed on it exclusively. Future queens continue to be nourished by this interesting product which is somehow responsible for their development into mature females.[2]

Because the resulting queens are much larger than worker bees, live ten times longer, and are highly fertile (worker bees are sterile), enthusiasts have long hoped that royal jelly might have beneficial effects when consumed or applied externally by human beings. The product is commercially available in a wide variety of forms, including ampules, capsules, creams, lotions, soap, and the like.

Various writers have claimed that royal jelly is especially effective: in halting or controlling the aging process—to nourish the skin and erase facial blemishes and wrinkles; also in cases of fatigue, depression, convalescence from illness, the "growing pains" of adolescence; and in preventing the signs of normal aging or even premature senility. As a general tonic for treating the menopause or male climacteric and to improve sexual performance, royal jelly supposedly has a general systemic action rather than any specific biological function.[3] The advertising brochure for a Chinese product also advocates its use in cases of liver disease, rheumatoid arthritis, anemia, phlebitis, gastric ulcer, degenerative conditions, and general mental or physical weakness.[4]

Although the chemistry of royal jelly is still not completely known, it has been extensively studied and found to contain protein, lipids, carbohydrates, fatty acids, and vitamins. The B vitamins were especially prominent, with pantothenic acid predominating. Tests have shown that royal jelly does possess some slight antibacterial activity; it can also affect the adrenal cortex and produce hyperglycemia (high blood sugar). An antitumor effect in mice has also been noted. But there is no evidence that the product has any estrogenic (female sex hormonal) activity, or that it affects the growth, longevity, or fertility of animals.[5]

As for its topical effectiveness in rejuvenating the skin, the results from one 3-month clinical study of 24 female patients are of interest. Ten women showed improvement, 10 experienced no change, and 4 showed symptoms of skin irritation.[6] These are equivocal results at best.

In view of the lack of evidence to support these claims of therapeutic usefulness, we can only agree with Dayan.[5] Any value in human beings is purely psychological (attributable to the placebo effect) and springs from the novelty and glamor of treatment with such an exotic product. One physiological effect of royal jelly is indisputable. It does have the ability to produce queens from ordinary bee larvae. Prudent readers will limit its use to that purpose. Those baldies in Budapest are still flat on top and so are their wallets!

REFERENCES

1. The Indianapolis Star, March 15, 1979, p. 1.
2. V. E. Tyler, L. R. Brady, and J. E. Robbers: Pharmacognosy, 8th Ed. Lea & Febiger, Philadelphia, 1981, p. 495.
3. S. S. Jones: Herbalist 4(10): 24–25, 1979.
4. Peking Royal Jelly, Peking Dietetic Preparation Manufactory, Peking, n.d.
5. A. D. Dayan: Journal of Pharmacy and Pharmacology 12: 377–383, 1960.
6. J. S. Jellinek: Formulation and Function of Cosmetics, John Wiley & Sons, New York, 1970, pp. 393–394.

RUE

Fresh leaves of the small, yellow-flowered, evergreen shrub, *Ruta graveolens* L. (family Rutaceae) emit a strongly disagreeable odor which, once smelled, will not be forgotten. Native to Europe, but naturalized and cultivated in the United States, this unpleasantly aromatic plant has been used since ancient times to prevent contagion (plague) and to repel insects as well as to heal their bites.[1] Dried rue leaves, which are less fragrant due to loss of much of their contained volatile oil, have also long been used as a folk remedy, particularly as an antispasmodic (to relieve cramps), calmative, emmenagogue (promotes the menstrual flow), and abortifacient.

Rue does contain a number of active constituents. A mixture of quinoline alkaloids, present in the herb to the extent of 1.4%, and especially one designated arborine, possess spasmolytic and abortifacient properties. Coumarin derivatives, a large number of which are present in the plant and in its volatile oil, also contribute appreciably to its spasmolytic properties.[2,3]

Unfortunately, these so-called furocoumarins, such as bergapten and xanthoxanthin, confer a significant toxicity especially on fresh rue, causing it to blister the skin following contact and exposure to sunlight (photosensitization).* An Indiana woman and her two young sons who rubbed fresh rue leaves on their exposed skin after reading about its insect repellant properties in a gardening magazine suffered from hives and large blisters (some 3 inches across) that required more than 2 weeks of treatment by a physician.[4] The fresh plant taken internally may result in gastric upsets, and Pahlow warns that these may also be caused by large doses of the dried leaves.[5] However, the toxicity of rue is much diminished on drying as a result of a decrease in the volatile oil content.

Several statements about rue in the current herbal literature need clarification: There is no evidence to support the assertion that any adverse symptoms from an overdose of the drug can be overcome by administering a small amount of goldenseal.[6] It is certainly doubtful that rubbing fresh rue leaves on the forehead will cure a headache,[7] but it is reasonably certain that this will

---

*See angelica for additional comments on the toxicity of these so-called psoralens.

result in a kind of dermatitis much worse than the original headache!

While there is little question about the antispasmodic action of rue, there is appreciable doubt about the utility and safety of the drug, especially in the fresh state. Medicinal use of the plant, fresh or dried, is not recommended for anybody, and under no circumstances should it be taken by pregnant women. Belief in rue as a valuable medicinal agent is as ridiculous as the belief that if the gunflints for a flintlock muzzle loader were boiled in a mixture of rue and vervain, the shot would hit its mark no matter how poor the aim of the marksman.[1]

REFERENCES

1. H. N. Moldenke and A. L. Moldenke: Plants of the Bible. Chronica Botanica Co., Waltham, Mass., 1952, p. 208.
2. P. H. List and L. Hörhammer, Eds.: Hagers Handbuch der Pharmazeutischen Praxis, 4th Ed. Vol. 6B. Springer-Verlag, Berlin, 1979, pp. 204–208.
3. A. Y. Leung: Encyclopedia of Common Natural Ingredients Used in Food, Drugs, and Cosmetics. John Wiley & Sons, New York, 1980, pp. 285–287.
4. J. Gengler: Gary Post Tribune, July 31, 1982, pp. A1, A3.
5. M. Pahlow: Das grosse Buch der Heilpflanzen. Gräfe und Unzer GmbH, Munich, 1979, pp. 266–267.
6. M. Tierra: The Way of Herbs. Unity Press, Santa Cruz, Calif., 1980, p. 113.
7. N. Coon: Using Plants for Healing, 2nd Ed. Rodale Press, Emmaus, Pa., 1979, p. 178.

SAGE

There is an old proverb:

> He that would live for aye,
> Must eat sage in May

which aptly summarizes the folkloric belief in the leaves of common garden sage as an almost magical cure-all. This well-known plant with its many branched stem, opposite hairy leaves, and blue, rarely pink or white, flowers is cultivated in the temperate parts of Europe and North America. Known by the scientific name *Salvia officinalis* L., it belongs to the mint family or Labiatae. Commercial samples are frequently adulterated with Greek sage, *Salvia triloba* L.

Keller lists more than 60 different ailments for which sage is claimed to be therapeutic.[1] Alphabetically, these range from aches to wounds and include such conditions as congealed blood, falling sickness (epilepsy), insomnia, measles, rheumatism, seasickness, venereal disease, and worms. There is really little need to elaborate on these, for if one consults a wide enough variety of modern herbals, it is highly probable that every sickness known to man will be listed as being cured by sage — plus a special ability to strengthen the nerves, quicken the senses and the memory, and promote longevity.[2]

On a more rational level, sage is taken extensively as a household remedy in Europe for several purposes: an aid in drying up the flow of mother's milk at the end of the nursing period; internally to reduce the secretion of saliva; and particularly as an anhidrotic (reduces or stops perspiration) to control the night sweats associated with diseases like tuberculosis. According to its supporters, various liquid preparations of sage relieve inflammations of the oral cavity and throat when used as a mouthwash or gargle.[3]

This last action on the mucous membranes is readily accounted for by sage's content of volatile oil and tannin. Its 1 to 2.8% of volatile oil, consisting mainly of α- and β-thujones, has been shown to possess antiseptic properties; its condensed catechin-type tannin acts as an astringent and also stimulates blood flow by its local irritant properties. These actions combine to make sage useful in treating mouth and throat irritations. Unfortunately, some of the other medicinal properties of sage are more controversial and not so readily explained.

However, clinical studies carried out on sage tincture and sage tea as early as 1896 demonstrated the drug's ability to suppress perspiration. This action was confirmed by repeated experiments conducted during the early decades of this century which showed that perspiration was reduced by about one-half, maximum effect being achieved in about 2–2 ½ hours. The activity is attributed to constituents in the volatile oil. A proprietary preparation of it, Salysat® is currently marketed in Germany as an anhidrotic.[4]

In 1939, experiments demonstrated estrogenic (female sex hormonal) activity following injection of sage extracts in mice. The compound(s) responsible for this effect remains unidentified. Furthermore, the relationship, if any, of this activity to the drug's purported ability to dry up the milk of nursing mothers is extremely unclear.

Other pharmacological investigations showed that administration of a decoction (boiled aqueous extract) of sage produced significant reduction of blood sugar in human subjects suffering from diabetes. The drug was particularly effective when taken on an empty stomach.[5]

All of these scientific studies would obviously confirm many of the uses of sage as a popular household remedy if it were not for an extensive investigation conducted in 1949 by H. B. J. van Rijn which cast doubt, or at least raised a real question, concerning them. Using small animals, he was unable to demonstrate any anhidrotic effect in sage, nor could he detect effects on blood pressure and respiration. In addition, he could not show any antibacterial action of the drug which also produced contradictory actions on various smooth muscles of the different organs (intestines and uterus). Finally, he did show a marked toxic effect of sage, probably attributable to its thujone-containing volatile oil.[6]

Details of the poisonous character of thujone are provided in the section on wormwood to come. Basically, it can cause both mental and physical deterioration when consumed in small amounts over a long period of time. Large doses can result in convulsions and loss of consciousness. We know that the plants containing it are not innocuous, so if van Rijn was right in this part of his study, he may also have been correct in his conclusion that sage, aside from its astringent action, is without medicinal value.

Even if it did have some therapeutic usefulness, sage cannot be recommended as a medicinal because of its high thujone content. Adding the leaves as a spice or flavoring agent in cooked foods is probably not critical since the heat involved apparently drives off most of the volatile thujone. Still, to be absolutely safe, we probably should reword that old adage a little to read:

"He that would live for aye,
Won't eat much sage in May—
Or any other month."

REFERENCES

1. M. S. Keller: Mysterious Herbs & Roots, Peace Press, Culver City, Calif., 1978, pp. 300–314.
2. M. Israel: Medical Herbalist 9: 173, 1936–37.
3. E. Steinegger and R. Hänsel: Lehrbuch der Pharmakognosie, 3rd Ed. Springer-Verlag, Berlin, 1972, pp. 446–447.
4. Rote Liste 1981, Editio Cantor KG, Aulendorf/Württ., 1981, index no. 31 287.
5. F. Berger: Handbuch der Drogenkunde, Vol. 2. Verlag Wilhelm Maudrich, Vienna, 1950, pp. 292–305.
6. H. B. J. van Rijn: Pharmaceutisch Weekblad 84: 337–343, 1949.

ST. JOHN'S WORT

Because *Hypericum perforatum* L., an aromatic perennial herb belonging to the family Hypericaceae, produces golden yellow flowers which seem to be particularly abundant on June 24, the day traditionally celebrated as the birthday of John the Baptist, the plant is commonly known as St. John's wort. Its overground parts (leaves and flowering tops) which are medicinally applied also begin to be harvested at about that time.[1] The plant is native to Europe but is found throughout the United States.

St. John's wort was known to such ancient authorities on medicinal plants as Dioscorides and Hippocrates; indeed it is described and recommended as a useful remedy in all of the herbals down through the Middle Ages. But like many plant drugs, it fell into disrepute in the late 19th century and was nearly forgotten. Quite recently, a tea prepared from the herb has acquired a renewed reputation, particularly in Europe, as an effective nerve tonic, useful in cases of anxiety, depression, and unrest. Users also value it internally as a diuretic and in the treatment of various conditions ranging from insomnia to gastritis.[2]

An olive oil extract of the fresh flowers of St. John's wort acquires a reddish color after standing in sunlight for several weeks. This so-called red oil is taken internally for the same conditions as is the tea, but it is also applied externally to relieve inflammation and promote healing. It is highly valued in the treatment of hemorrhoids.[3,4]

Chemical investigations have detected a number of constituents in St. John's wort including about 1% of a volatile oil and approximately 10% of tannin. The latter compound probably exerts some wound-healing effects through its astringent and protein-precipitating actions. Much of the activity reported for the plant is due, however, to the presence of hypericin, a reddish dianthrone pigment. Very small doses of hypericin produce a tonic and tranquilizing action in human beings, apparently by increasing capillary blood flow.[5] Reducing capillary fragility is another recorded action of the compound.[6]

Unfortunately, hypericin may exert another action which is much less desirable. The compound is known to induce a kind of photosensitivity characterized by dermatitis of the skin and inflammation of the mucous membranes on exposure to direct sunlight.[7] While this seldom happens with normal doses of St. John's wort, those who take the herb for extended periods should be aware of the possibility and discontinue usage if such symptoms occur.

REFERENCES

1. H.-J. Weidinger: Heilkräuter: anbauen – sammeln – nützen – schützen. Verlag Fritz Molden, Vienna, 1981, pp. 114 – 117.
2. P. Schmidsberger: Knaurs Buch der Heilpflanzen. Droemer Knaur, Munich, 1980, pp. 103 – 106.
3. M. Pahlow: Heilpflanzen heute. Gräfe und Unzer GmbH, Munich, n.d., pp. 65 – 66.
4. G. Mihailescu and A. Mihailescu: Pflanzen helfen heil. Biblio Verlagsgesellschaft mbH, Munich, 1979, pp. 56 – 57.
5. K. Daniel: Die Pharmazie 6: 131, 1951.
6. F. Galla and G. Verza: Quaderni fitoterapia (Milan) No. 8: 1 – 47, 1957.
7. P. H. List and L. Hörhammer, Eds.: Hagers Handbuch der Pharmazeutischen Praxis, 4th Ed., Vol. 5. Springer-Verlag, Berlin, 1976, pp. 214 – 217.

SARSAPARILLA

The roots of several woody climbing plants native to Central and South America constitute the drug sarsaparilla. All of them are species of the genus *Smilax* belonging to the family Liliaceae. Included are S. *aristolochiaefolia* Miller known as Mexican sarsaparilla, S. *regelii* Killip et Morton commonly referred to as Honduran sarsaparilla, S. *febrifuga* Kunth or Ecuadorian sarsaparilla, as well as other undetermined species of *Smilax*.[1]

After it was introduced to Europe from the New World in the mid-16th century, the drug was valued primarily as a treatment for syphilis.[2] This reputation, disguised under the terms "alterative" or "blood purifier," continued in medical circles well into the present century. As Mrs. Alice West of Jefferson, West Virginia, put it in an early-day patent medicine advertisement[3]:

> I was all run down before I began to take Ayer's Sarsaparilla, but now I am gaining strength every day. I intend using the Sarsaparilla till my health is perfectly restored.

Of course, this puts a slightly different light on the white-hatted cowboy hero who always strode to the bar in the Saturday afternoon B movie and, shunning the alcoholic beverages which were being drunk by the black-hatted villains, calmly said, "Give me a bottle of Sarsaparilla."

Sarsaparilla contains a mixture of saponins derived mainly from sarsapogenin and smilagenin.[1] The saponins have a strong diuretic action as well as some diaphoretic, expectorant, and laxative properties. In addition, the plant material is a moderately useful flavoring agent. Neither the whole drug nor its contained saponins is effective in the treatment of syphilis or as a "blood purifier."

REFERENCES

1. V. E. Tyler, L. R. Brady, and J. E. Robbers: Pharmacognosy. 8th Ed. Lea & Febiger, Philadelphia, 1981, p. 495–496.
2. F. A. Flückiger and D. Hanbury: Pharmacographia. Macmillan, London, 1879, pp. 703–712.
3. A. Hechtlinger: The Great Patent Medicine Era. Grosset & Dunlap, New York, 1970, p. 76.

SASSAFRAS

"Fill me with sassafras, nurse,
And juniper juice!
Let me see if I'm still any use!"
Donald Robert Perry Marquis
"Spring Ode"

Sassafras is a plant whose virtues are uniformly praised by modern herbalists. A tea prepared from the root bark of this native American tree, *Sassafras albidum* (Nutt.) Nees of the family Lauraceae, is widely recommended as a spring tonic and "blood thinner." The root bark was being used to treat fevers by the natives of Florida prior to 1512 and formed one of the earliest exports of the New World. It still enjoys a considerable reputation as a stimulant, antispasmodic, sudorific (sweat producer), depurative ("purifier") and as treatment for rheumatism, skin diseases, syphilis, typhus, dropsy (fluid accumulation), and so on.[1]

Much of the persistent reputation of sassafras may no doubt be attributed to its pleasant taste and aroma. It contains up to 9% of a volatile oil which, in turn, consists of about 80% safrole. For years it was a valued flavoring agent in root beer and similar beverages. But as a result of research conducted in the early 1960's, safrole was recognized as a carcinogenic agent in rats and mice.[2] Both sassafras oil and safrole were prohibited by the FDA from use as flavors or food additives.

Unfortunately, sassafras continued to be collected, used, sold, and written about as an herbal remedy. No one really knows just how harmful it is to human beings, but it has been estimated that one cup of strong sassafras tea could contain as much as 200 mg. of safrole, more than four times the minimal amount believed hazardous to man if consumed on a regular basis.[3]

Some manufacturers, recognizing the attractive flavor and aroma of sassafras, have attempted to overcome its toxicity by preparing a safrole-free extract of the root bark. Such efforts were probably doomed to failure from the start since safrole is the major component responsible for the desirable odor and taste of the plant. However, an even more serious drawback has been revealed. Recent studies have shown that even safrole-free sassafras produced tumors in two-thirds of the animals treated with it.[4] Apparently other constituents in addition to safrole are responsible for part of the root bark's carcinogenic activity.

As a matter of fact, a question was raised about the carcinogenicity of safrole in man by a 1977 study carried out by toxicologists in Switzerland.[5] They were unable to demonstrate the formation 1'-hydroxysafrole, the metabolite actually responsible for safrole's cancer-producing effect, when small amounts of safrole were given by mouth to human volunteers. On the other hand, this so-called proximate carcinogen was detected in the urine of rats when safrole was fed to those animals. The finding suggests that the toxicity of safrole in man and in small animals may differ.

However, the doses of safrole given to the human subjects in the Swiss study were extremely small (maximum 1.655 mg.), and this may account for the failure of the human subjects to metabolize it to 1'-hydroxysafrole. More studies are definitely necessary before any final conclusion can be reached regarding the safety of sassafras as an herbal remedy.

An overriding consideration in this entire matter of the safety and efficacy of sassafras is that the plant material has no really significant medical or therapeutic utility. Sassafras oil, in common with a large number of volatile oils, does possess some mild counterirritant properties on external application, but beyond these, none of the claims of its supporters has been documented in the modern medical literature. In spite of its pleasant flavor and its folkloric reputation as a useful tonic, prudent people will avoid this drug because of its potentially harmful qualities.

Modern scientific evidence compels us to revise Marquis' verse:

> Shun the sassafras, nurse,
> Bring juniper juice!
> It's one herb I can still misuse!

REFERENCES

1. J. U. Lloyd: Origin and History of All the Pharmacopeial Vegetable Drugs, Chemicals and Preparations, Vol. 1. The Caxton Press, Cincinnati, 1921, pp. 289–297.
2. IARC Monographs on the Evaluation of the Carcinogenic Risk of Chemicals to Man 1: 169–174, 1972.
3. A. B. Segelman, F. P. Segelman, J. Karliner, and D. Sofia: Journal of the American Medical Association 236: 477, 1976.
4. G. J. Kapadia, E. B. Chung, B. Ghosh, Y. N. Shukla, S. P. Basak, J. F. Morton, and S. N. Pradhan: Journal of the National Cancer Institute 60: 683–686, 1978.
5. M. S. Benedetti, A Malnoë, and L. Broillet: Toxicology 7: 69–83, 1977.

SAVORY

Ancient herbals commonly mention two savories: summer, which consists of the overgrown portions of *Satureja hortensis* L., and winter, obtained from *S. montana* L. These two aromatic members of the mint (Labiatae) family are small, widely cultivated garden plants with narrow leaves and pale lavender, pink, or white flowers. Summer savory, which is more highly prized as a spice and as a folk medicine, is an annual; winter savory is a perennial. For hundreds of years, both have enjoyed a reputation as sex drugs.[1] Summer savory was believed to increase desire (act as an aphrodisiac), and winter savory was believed to decrease the sex drive (anaphrodisiac). It is easy to see why summer savory became the more popular herb.

In modern folk medicine, summer savory is currently believed to benefit the entire digestive system. According to its believers, the herb acts as a carminative, an antiflatulent, an appetite stimulant, and also works in diarrhea. A tea prepared from the herb is considered beneficial as an expectorant and cough remedy.[2] One very interesting use of the tea in Europe is for excessive thirst in diabetics.[3] Many other therapeutic applications are listed by various herbalists, but most of these (for example, improving vision and curing deafness) are so farfetched that they are not worth repeating.[4]

An extremely valuable use of summer savory is as a spice. It gives an excellent flavor to beans and other legumes.[1] In fact, its German name is *Bohnenkraut* or bean herb. Both savories, as well as the aromatic volatile oils obtained from them, are much used in flavoring various kinds of sausages.

Summer savory contains from 0.3 to 2% of a volatile oil consisting of about 30% carvacrol, 20–30% p-cymene, and lesser amounts of numerous other constituents. The plant also contains 4 to 8.5% of tannin.[3] Other compounds have been identified in the herb, but none has any noticeable physiological activity.

Because of its content of carvacrol and p-cymene, the volatile oil confers a mild antiseptic property on summer savory. This apparently combines with the astringent effect of the contained tannin to make the plant of some little value in simple diarrhea. The oil is probably fairly effectual, especially when combined with hot water in the form of a tea, for minor throat irritations and mild digestive upsets. Besides, it tastes good and is relatively harmless, at least in moderate amounts. Summer savory is certainly a pleasant herb; just don't expect too much from it.

REFERENCES

1. M. S. Keller: Mysterious Herbs & Roots. Peace Press, Culver City, Calif., 1978, pp. 316–325.
2. M. Pahlow: Das grosse Buch der Heilpflanzen. Gräfe und Unzer GmbH, Munich, 1979, pp. 93–97.
3. P. H. List and L. Hörhammer, Eds: Hagers Handbuch der Pharmazeutischen Praxis, 4th Ed., Vol. 6B. Springer-Verlag, Berlin, 1979, pp. 295–299.
4. M. Grieve: A Modern Herbal, Vol. 2. Dover Publications, New York, 1971, pp. 718–719.

SAW PALMETTO

If you bought a small paperback book for $2.00 and found a paragraph in it devoted to a berry which, taken regularly, would increase the size of underdeveloped female breasts, and also build sexual vigor, increase sperm production, reverse atrophy of the testes and mammary glands, and relieve catarrhal soreness of the genitourinary system, you might be tempted to try the berries—if, of course you had these problems.[1] You might even drink, three times a day, a tea made from the saw palmetto berries, and as one person did after some time, write your syndicated pharmacy columnist to find out why it had not become necessary to buy a bigger bra.[2]

The berries responsible for this true-to-life scenario are the ripe fruits, fresh or more often partially dried, of *Serenoa repens* (Bartr.) Small, also known as *S. serrulata* (Michx.) Nichols. Commonly called saw palmetto or sabal, the plant which produces these dusky red to brownish black berries is a fan palm (family Palmae), 6 to 10 feet tall, with leaf clusters 2 to 2.5 feet across, each consisting of 20 or more leaf blades, and each blade ending in two sharp points. Growing in sandy soil from South Carolina to Florida and west to Texas, the plant forms great colonies in the wild. Commercial supplies of the berries come from the area around Cape Canaveral, Florida.[3]

During the first half of this century, saw palmetto was frequently used in conventional medicine, mostly as a mild diuretic and as therapy for chronic cystitis; it was also considered good for enlargement of the prostate. The active constituent was supposed to be a volatile oil, but physicians began to question saw palmetto's efficacy, and in 1950, it was deleted from the listing of official drugs in *The National Formulary*.

Then during the 1960's, investigators found relatively high concentrations of free and bound sitosterols in the dried berries. Various plant extracts as well as pure β-sitosterol, which was also isolated, exhibited estrogenic activity when *injected* into immature female mice. Although the activity was found to be relatively high compared to other estrogens isolated from plants, it was rather low in comparison to the female sex hormones themselves. A saw palmetto extract was only about 1/10,000 as potent as estradiol, and even pure β-sitosterol was less than $\frac{1}{10}$ as strong.[4]

But it must be kept in mind that these comparisons were made in experiments where the drugs were injected under the skin of the animals; they were not given by mouth. The sitosterols are poorly absorbed from the gastrointestinal tract and as a matter of fact, are administered orally not for their estrogenic activity but to compete with cholesterol for absorption sites in the intestine in order to treat atherosclerosis.[5] When the relative insolubility of β-sitosterol in water is added to this poor intestinal absorption phenomenon, it is easy to see that a cup of saw palmetto tea contains about as much real estrogenic activity as a cup of hot water. It would be convenient if the facts were different, for some of the advertised actions of the plant (breast development, treatment of enlarged prostate) could be explained on the basis of estrogenic activity, but they are not. Other effects, such as improved sexual vigor (at least in the male) and increased sperm production would be exactly the opposite of those which might be expected of an estrogen.

Nevertheless, authors of counterculture publications, apparently misled by their incomplete understanding of the scientific literature, added the fictitious property of breast development to the actions already attributed to saw palmetto.[1,6] This myth reached the "health food" stores and is now so firmly established as part of modern herbal lore that it will probably require years of disappointment on the part of hopeful but gullible users before it can be eradicated. At present, we can only reemphasize that saw palmetto definitely does not increase the size of mammary glands and is of doubtful value for any therapeutic purpose whatsoever.

Still, nothing is entirely worthless. In 1969, federally sponsored research showed that saw palmetto was one of three plants, out of a group of 30 tested, that provided all of the nutrients necessary for prolonging the lives of mosquitoes.[7]Some insects may thus benefit from it, even if picnickers and underdeveloped females won't.

REFERENCES

1. A. Gottlieb: Sex Drugs and Aphrodisiacs. High Times/Level Press, New York and San Francisco, 1974, p. 64.
2. J. Graedon: The Indianapolis Star, April 15, 1981, p. 18.
3. H. W. Youngken: Textbook of Pharmacognosy, 6th Ed. The Blakiston Co., Philadelphia, 1948, pp. 168–171.

4. M. I. Elghamry and R. Hänsel: Experientia 25: 828–829, 1969.
5. V. E. Tyler, L. R. Brady, and J. E. Robbers: Pharmacognosy, 8th Ed. Lea & Febiger, Philadelphia, 1981, p. 168.
6. M. J. Superweed: Herbal Aphrodisiacs. Stone Kingdom Syndicate, San Francisco, 1971, p. 5.
7. R. S. Paterson, B. J. Smittle, and R. T. DeNeve: Journal of Economic Entomology 62: 1455–1458, 1969.

SCHISANDRA

Perhaps the newest of the old drugs resurrected by the American herbal medicine industry is schisandra, or schizandra, the dried ripe fruit of *Schisandra chinensis* (Turcz.) Baill., a tree native to China. Its ancient folkloric use there was as an antiseptic, astringent, tonic and the like. During the last decade or so, Chinese doctors began using the drug to treat hepatitis, and a few studies have been done of its potential for liver-protective effects and the nature of its active constituents.

Western herbal advocates now acclaim schisandra as an "adaptogen," an agent supposedly capable of increasing the body's resistance to disease, stress, and other debilitating processes. Schisandra is said to "increase energy, replenish and nourish viscera, improve vision, boost muscular activity and affect the energy cells of the entire body."[1] One marketer claims that its schisandra product can "help to combat damage that can lead to premature aging." Another notes that its product is "capable of providing a more healthy, active and longer lifespan." Schisandra ads also claim that it is effective against premenstrual syndrome, stimulates immune defenses, balances body function, normalizes body systems, boosts recovery after surgery, protects against radiation, counteracts the effects of sugar, optimizes energy in times of stress, increases stamina, protects against motion sickness, normalizes blood sugar and blood pressure, reduces high cholesterol, shields against infection, improves the health of the adrenals, energizes RNA—DNA molecules to rebuild cells, and "produces energy comparable to that of a young athlete."

Limited studies of schisandra's effects have been carried out in small animals. An investigation conducted by L. Volicer and colleagues in Czechoslovakia in 1966 noted that the drug had a stimulating effect in low doses, but this was reversed with large doses. These actions are similar to those of nicotine.[2]

The constituents responsible for the liver-protective effects of schisandra are apparently lignans—molecules composed of two phenylpropanoid units. More than 30 of these have been isolated from schisandra, some 22 of which were tested in 1984 by the Japanese investigator H. Hikino for their ability to reduce the cytotoxic effects of carbon tetrachloride and galactosamine on cultured rat liver cells.[3] Most were found effective, and some were quite active. However, when galactosamine was used as a cytotoxic agent, the protective effects of the lignans were reduced at higher doses. Dr. Hikino concluded that the lignans of schisandra were themselves toxic to the liver when administered in large doses over a long period of time.

Subsequently, Japanese investigators have investigated the mechanism by which two of the lignans, wuweizisu C and gomisin A, exert their liver protective effects. They found that both compounds functioned as antioxidants, thereby preventing the lipid peroxidation produced by harmful substances such as carbon tetrachloride. Since lipid peroxidation leads to the formation of harmful lesions in the liver, the two compounds did indeed exert a protective influence.[4]

However, the reported evidence to date on the stimulatory and liver-protective role of schisandra is somewhat equivocal and certainly preliminary in nature. To determine whether schisandra has practical value as a drug, long-term studies of safety and effectiveness at various dose levels — first in animals and ultimately in human beings — are definitely needed.

REFERENCES

1. R. D. Marconi: Let's Grow Younger. Scientific Nutrition Press, Seal Beach, Calif., 1983, pp. 9–10.
2. L. Volicer, M. Šramka, I. Janků, R. Čapek, R. Smetana, and V. Ditteová: Archives Internationales de Pharmacodynamie et de therapie 163: 249–262, 1966.
3. H. Hikino: In Natural Products and Drug Development, P. Krogsgaard-Larsen, S. B. Christensen, and H. Kofod, Eds. Munksgaard, Copenhagen, 1984, pp. 374–389.
4. Y. Kiso, M. Tohkin, H. Hikino, Y. Ikeya, and H. Taguchi: Planta Medica 51: 331–334, 1985.

SCULLCAP

That a nearly worthless and essentially inactive plant material could be recommended in a 1970 publication[1] as a "useful tranquilizing herb" and praised in an herbal revised in 1975[2] as "one of the finest nervines [tranquilizers] ever discovered," says much about the gullibility of human beings. Nevertheless, such is the case with scullcap, the overground parts of the plant Scutellaria lateriflora L., a member of the family Labiatae. This plant is native to the United States, but several different species have been employed in medicine; S. baicalensis Georgi, a native of East Asia, is the one commonly utilized in Europe. All are rather similar, erect, perennial herbs which reach a height of about two feet.

Scullcap was introduced into American medicine in 1773 by Dr. Lawrence Van Derveer who used it to treat cases of hydrophobia. The name mad-dog herb stems from this. Subsequently, it came to be utilized primarily for its reputed tonic, tranquilizing, and antispasmodic effects. As such, it was a common ingredient in many proprietary remedies for "female weakness." The drug was officially in The United States Pharmacopeia from 1863 to 1916 and then in The National Formulary until it was dropped in 1947.[3]

In 1916 Pilcher tested an extract of scullcap for its effect on the contractility of the excised guinea pig uterus and found its slightly depressant properties to be the least active of the drugs tested. Since it had no effect in normal doses on the uterus of living animals, he concluded the drug lacked therapeutic value.[4] In 1957, Kurnakov studied the effects of extracts of two other species of scullcap, S. galericulata L. and S. scordiifolia Fisch. ex Schrank, in various small animals. Neither had any effect on blood pressure in cats or rabbits, nor did they depress the central nervous system in frogs. They also failed to exert any antispasmodic activity.[5] The report by Usow, a year later, that a tincture of S. baicalensis produced a long-lasting decline in blood pressure in dogs is contradictory and requires verification.[6]

Various species of Scutellaria contain a number of flavonoid pigments, including baicalein, scutellarein, and wogonin which might be thought responsible for the antispasmodic effects attributed to the whole drug. Tests in mice showed that baicalein had no detectable antispasmodic activity while that of wogonin was very slight, about one-fifth that of papaverine hydrochloride.[7]

Nearly forty years ago, at a time when scullcap was still officially recognized in *The National Formulary*, Wood and Osol aptly summarized its virtues or, rather, lack thereof[8]:

> Scullcap is as destitute of medicinal properties as a plant may well be, not even being aromatic. When taken internally, it produces no very obvious effects, and probably is of no remedial value. . . .

REFERENCES

1. M. J. Superweed: Herbal Highs. Stone Kingdom Syndicate, San Francisco, 1970, pp. 15–16.
2. R. C. Wren and R. W. Wren: Potter's New Cyclopaedia of Botanical Drugs and Preparations, New Ed. Health Science Press, Hengiscote, England, 1975, p. 274.
3. E. P. Claus: Pharmacognosy, 3rd Ed. Lea & Febiger, Philadelphia, 1956, pp. 219–220.
4. T. Sollman: A Manual of Pharmacology, 7th Ed. W. B. Saunders, Philadelphia, 1948, p. 406.
5. B. A. Kurnakov: Farmakologiya i Toksikologiya (Moscow) 206: 79–80, 1957.
6. P. H. List and L. Hörhammer, Eds.: Hagers Handbuch der Pharmazeutischen Praxis, 4th Ed., Vol. 6B. Springer-Verlag, Berlin, 1979, p. 340.
7. S. Shibata, M. Harada, and W. Budidarmo: Yakugaku Zasshi 80: 620–624, 1960.
8. H. C. Wood, Jr. and A. Osol: The Dispensatory of the United States of America, 23rd Ed. J. B. Lippincott, Philadelphia, 1943, pp. 965–966.

SENEGA SNAKEROOT

Plant roots often assume a twisted, tortuous shape, so the name snakeroot is an apt one. Unfortunately, it is applied to so many different species (some of which are listed in Chapter 2), that without a modifier the term is meaningless. Senega snakeroot, seneca snakeroot, or just plain senega refers to the yellow root of *Polygala senega* L., a perennial herb (family Polygonaceae) with small white flowers, native to the woodlands of eastern North America from southern Canada to South Carolina.[1]

It was one of the new remedies introduced into medicine after the discovery of America where the Seneca Indians valued it as a cure for rattlesnake bite. Although this usage was probably based purely on the "Doctrine of Signatures," senega subsequently enjoyed great popularity as a nauseant expectorant and was a common ingredient in syrups and similar preparations for coughs and colds. The drug's popularity declined in recent years and in 1960, it was dropped from *The National Formulary*. Modern herbalists continue to praise its virtues as an expectorant, diaphoretic (promotes perspiration), sialogogue (increases the flow of saliva), and emetic. It is said to be particularly good for asthma and bronchitis.[2]

Fresh senega snakeroot has a pleasant odor reminiscent of wintergreen due to its content of approximately 0.1% methyl salicylate. The active ingredient, however, is a complex mixture of triterpenoid saponins in the root in a concentration ranging from 6 to 10%.[3] The saponins act by local irritation on the lining of the stomach, thus causing nausea which in turn stimulates both bronchial secretions and the sweat glands. Large doses cause vomiting and purging.[1]

There is no question about the effectiveness of senega snakeroot as an expectorant. It continues to be used in Europe as an ingredient in various syrups, lozenges, and tea mixtures for controlling coughs and related throat irritations. If it is utilized in any of these forms, one must be careful to follow the recommended dosage, or stomach upsets will follow. For this and other reasons, the drug is simply not included in any commercial preparations in the United States. The *Handbook of Nonprescription Drugs* lists nine pages of cough syrups with their ingredients, none of which contains senega as an expectorant,[4] so we can only conclude that safer and more effective cough treatments exist. If you need an expectorant, it is probably best to use something other than senega snakeroot.

REFERENCES

1. A. Osol and G. E. Farrar, Jr.: The Dispensatory of the United States of America, 24th Ed. J. B. Lippincott, Philadelphia, 1947, pp. 1018–1019.
2. L. Veninga and B. R. Zaricor: Goldenseal/Etc. Ruka Publications, Santa Cruz, Calif., 1976, pp. 167–169.
3. P. H. List and L. Hörhammer, Eds.: Hagers Handbuch der Pharmazeutischen Praxis, 4th Ed., Vol. 6A. Springer-Verlag, Berlin, 1977, pp. 802–807.
4. Handbook of Nonprescription Drugs, 8th Ed. American Pharmaceutical Association, Washington, D.C., 1986, pp. 153–161.

SENNA

"There was an Old Man of Vienna, who lived
  upon tincture of senna;
When that did not agree he took chamomile
tea,
That nasty Old Man of Vienna."
              Edward Lear
              The Book of Nonsense

It is possible that the Old Man of Vienna who found senna so disagreeable was the forerunner of the modern housewife who had a similar experience with the drug. Tired of the customary caffeine beverages and seeking an alternative hot drink, she selected a package of senna, unlabeled as to its use, from the shelf of a "health food" store. This beverage proved to be a different-tasting one, so she drank several strong cups of it during breakfast the next morning. After spending that afternoon and evening in the bathroom and in bed suffering from diarrhea accompanied by nausea, intense griping, and subsequent dehydration, she called her physician. He told her what she had already learned from the sad experience. Senna is a potent cathartic and in measured amounts, a common ingredient in many proprietary laxatives.

Is this minor tragedy exaggerated or farfetched? Not at all! Several similar cases are cited in the literature.[1]

Senna or senna leaves are actually the dried leaflets of two species of *Cassia: C. acutifolia* Delile, known as Alexandria senna, and *C. angustifolia* Vahl, known as Tinnevelly senna. Both plants are small shrubs of the family Leguminosae. The former species grows along the Nile in Egypt and Sudan, and the latter is extensively cultivated in southern and eastern India. Senna was introduced into European medicine in the 9th or 10th century by the Arabs; its use as a native drug apparently antedates written records.[2]

The centuries-old practice of senna as a cathartic drug is based on its content of so-called dianthrone glycosides (1.5 to 3.0%), principally sennosides A and B with lesser amounts of sennosides C and D as well as other closely related compounds.[3] While it is certainly possible to take senna in the form of a tea prepared from 1 to 2 teaspoons of leaves, it may prove difficult to adjust the dosage of such an unstandardized preparation. Consequently, many consumers will prefer to select one of the many over-the-counter syrups, tablets, or similar products containing standardized amounts of active principles along with appropriate directions for use. Such preparations often contain added aromatic materials which somewhat modify the undesirable nauseant and griping effects of senna.[4]

In any case, remember that senna is a potent cathartic drug, not just a different-tasting tea. Habitual dosing with this or any other anthraquinone-containing laxative should be avoided or excessive irritation of the colon may result.[5]

REFERENCES

1. Anon.: Morbidity and Mortality Weekly Report 27:248–249,1978.
2. V. E. Tyler, L. R. Brady, and J. E. Robbers: Pharmacognosy, 8th Ed. Lea & Febiger, Philadelphia, 1981, pp. 64–66,498.
3. A. Y. Leung: Encyclopedia of Common Natural Ingredients Used in Food, Drugs, and Cosmetics. John Wiley & Sons, New York, 1980, pp. 297–299.
4. M. Grieve: A Modern Herbal, Vol. 2. Dover Publications, New York, 1971, pp. 734–737.
5. M. Pahlow: Das grosse Buch der Heilpflanzen. Gräfe und Unzer GmbH, Munich, 1979, pp. 426–427.

SPIRULINA

A favorite theme of futuristic fiction is mankind's struggle for survival on an overpopulated planet where people are reduced to eating mostly food prepared from cultivated algae in order to get adequate nourishment. But fact has a way of catching up with even the most imaginative fiction, so in 1987 (George Orwell of 1984 fame must be smiling) we see advertisements for the blue-green alga spirulina—one hundred 500 mg. tablets for about $6.00 or $7.00, the same size capsules or chewable wafers slightly higher.

Spirulina Turpin is a genus of blue-green algae belonging to the family Oscillatoriaceae of the division Cyanophyta.[1] There are numerous species, and the commercially available products are ordinarily not identified as to source. However, Switzer notes that two species are currently utilized: Spirulina maxima, cultivated in Mexico and S. platensis, cultivated in Thailand and California.[2]

Spirulina has for years been used as a food by natives of Africa and Mexico. Collected from the bottoms of seasonally dried-up ponds and shallow waters in the north of Lake Chad, where it has long been eaten by the African natives, it is known as dihe.[3] Early inhabitants of Tenochtitlán, the present-day Mexico City, also collected a blue-green alga of unknown identity (but presumably a Spirulina species) from nearby lakes which they found palatable. They called it tecuitlatl.[4] Much of the current commercial supply of spirulina comes from Lake Texcoco in Mexico, but the alga is also cultivated and harvested both in Thailand and in California.

Touted as the "super food of the future," spirulina is said to contain 50 to 70% of highly digestible protein containing all of the essential amino acids. It is also reputed to have twice as much vitamin B_{12} as liver, in addition to many other B vitamins, vitamins A and E, and minerals. Low in fat, with a mild and palatable flavor—like bean sprouts—spirulina has an intense green color which many consumers find objectionable.[5]

In addition to its food value, spirulina is called a "safe diet pill" and an exciting new way to lose weight safely and quickly. This is based on the alga's content of the amino acid phenylalanine which, according to one theory, affects the appetite center of the brain. Another theory is that eating spirulina raises the blood sugar concentration enough to influence the same hunger center of the brain, causing it to suppress hunger pangs.[6] Spirulina enthusiasts also say it's effective treatment for diabetes, hepatitis, cirrhosis of the liver, anemia, stress, pancreatitis, cataracts, glaucoma, ulcers, and loss of hair.[7]

Tests in rats have shown that a commercial spirulina preparation consisting of 50–70% protein, 4–7% moisture, 6.4–9% ash (minerals), and 13–16.5% carbohydrates was able to be the sole dietary source of protein for these animals.[8] The alga does contain protein with a satisfactory makeup of amino acids although the sulfur-containing ones, methionine and cystine, tend to be limiting.[9] Depending on the species, dried spirulina does contain between 0.5 and 2 μg. (microgram) per gram of vitamin B_{12}.[10] However, selective assay procedures suggest that more than 80% of the "vitamin B_{12}" in spirulina is, in fact, analogues of the vitamin which have no vitamin B_{12} activity in humans. This very low level of activity in spirulina compares to 0.2 – 1.8 μg. of the vitamin contained in 1 gram of liver.[11] The adult daily requirement of vitamin B_{12} is 5 to 6 μg.

Granting that spirulina may be an acceptable source of protein, the question then arises if it is an economical one. Assuming the present minimum price of $6.00 for one hundred 500 mg. tablets, then spirulina costs 12¢ per gram. If its protein content is a maximal 70%, then 1 gram of spirulina protein costs 17¢. Compare this with roast beef which, depending on the cut, may cost about $2.50 per pound, equivalent to just over ½ cent per gram. Considering its protein content to average 33%, then one gram of beef protein costs slightly more than 1.5 cents or about one-tenth the cost of spirulina protein! The alga is certainly not an economical food, and many will prefer the taste of roast beef, especially at one-tenth the price.

Does spirulina have anything else to offer? The vitamins and minerals it contains are easily obtained from other, more economical food sources. What about its effectiveness as an appetite suppressant? Any digestible carbohydrate-containing food will cause an increase in blood sugar and a corresponding reduction in hunger. Certainly there are more economical sources of carbohydrate than spirulina. There is no evidence to support the claim that phenylalanine is especially effective in reducing the appetite, and even if it were, that amino acid is readily available from a wide variety of more economical protein sources. In 1979, a Food and Drug Administration Advisory Panel reviewed spirulina and found no reliable scientific data to demonstrate that it is a safe and effective appetite suppressant.[12]

As for claims that spirulina is a kind of miracle cure for everything from diabetes to hair loss, examination of the evidence in supporting such assertions reveals that it is insubstantial at best. A lot more clinical evidence must be obtained before any such contention can be accepted . . . for example, the study on reduction of hair loss was carried out on one patient!

If the science-fiction writers are right, it may someday be necessary for human beings to eat blue-green algae in order to exist. Fortunately, that day has not yet arrived. With meat and other protein sources readily available at a mere fraction of the cost of spirulina, consuming an alga which offers no clear nutritional or therapeutic advantages seems neither useful nor rational.

REFERENCES

1. G. M. Smith: The Fresh-Water Algae of the United States. McGraw-Hill, New York, 1950, pp. 573–574.
2. L. Switzer: Spirulina, 3rd Ed. Proteus Corp., Berkeley, Calif., 1980.
3. J. Leónard: Nature 209: 126–128, 1966.
4. W. V. Farrar: Nature 211: 341–342, 1966.
5. H. N. Cole: Herbalist New Health 6(4): 15, 19, 1981.
6. R. G. Smith: National Enquirer, June 2, 1981, p. 23.
7. C. Hills, Ed.: The Secrets of Spirulina. University of the Trees, Boulder Creek, Calif., 1980.
8. A. Contreras, D. C. Herbert, B. G. Grubbs, and I. L. Cameron: Nutrition, Reports International 19: 749–763, 1979.
9. G. Clement: Revue de l'Institut Pasteur de Lyon 4: 103–114, 1971.
10. V. Herbert and G. Drivas: Journal of the American Medical Association 248: 3096–3097, 1982.
11. P. H. List and L. Hörhammer, Eds.: Hagers Handbuch der Pharmazeutischen Praxis, 4th Ed., Vol. 2. Springer-Verlag, Berlin, 1969, p. 690.
12. Anon.: Pharmacy Practice 16: 82, 1981.

TANSY

Most people tend to think of chrysanthemums as purely ornamental plants, but one species, *Chrysanthemum vulgare* (L.) Bernh., also known as *Tanacetum vulgare* L., family Compositae, has a long history in folk medicine. This strongly aromatic herb, which reaches a height of up to 3 feet and produces bright yellow flowers, is native to Europe but is naturalized and widely cultivated in the United States.

The dried leaves and flowering tops of tansy have been employed, usually in the form of a tea, as an anthelmintic (expels worms), tonic, stimulant, and emmenagogue (promotes menstrual flow — often a euphemism for promoting abortion). Tansy also makes a flavoring in cakes and puddings, especially those eaten at Easter. And it enjoys a considerable reputation as an insect repellent, especially for flies.[1]

Fresh tansy yields between 0.12% and 0.18% volatile oil which is extremely variable in its chemical composition, depending upon the specific source plants utilized. Indeed, scientists indicate that a number of chemical races of tansy exist which perpetuate their own distinctive composition of the oil, just as other plants breed true for flower color or a similar more noticeable characteristic. It is generally agreed that the physiological actions attributed to the plant mainly come from the thujone content of the oil.[2] But some tansy oils are entirely free of thujone, and others contain as much as 95% of that compound.[3] This composition is determined by the genetic makeup of the plant and is not appreciably influenced by environmental factors. Thus the effect of any tansy preparation will be dependent on the chemical race represented, since this determines the thujone content of the contained volatile oil. Without subjecting a specific plant sample to an analysis for thujone, it is impossible to estimate the proper dosage for a tansy preparation.

Moreover, as mentioned in the discussion on wormwood, thujone is a relatively toxic compound, capable of inducing both convulsions and psychotic effects in human beings. There are far more effective and much safer medicines than the thujone-containing tansy for expelling and destroying intestinal worms — the principal use of the plant in folk medicine.[4] In this enlightened era, there is absolutely no reason to utilize a potentially dangerous, toxic material of this sort as an emmenagogue-abortifacient. As a matter of fact, since far more effective insect repellents are readily available, there is no real reason to use tansy for anything. Well, perhaps there is just one. Tansy is used as a flavoring agent in certain alcoholic beverages, including Chartreuse, but the resulting product must be thujone-free.

REFERENCES

1. M. Grieve: A Modern Herbal, Vol. 2. Dover Publications, New York, 1971, pp. 789–790.
2. P. H. List and L. Hörhammer, Eds.: Hagers Handbuch der Pharmazeutischen Praxis, 4th Ed., Vol. 3. Springer-Verlag, Berlin, 1972, pp. 902–905.
3. E. Stahl and G. Schmitt: Archiv der Pharmazie 297: 385–391, 1964.
4. M. Pahlow: Das grosse Buch der Heilpflanzen. Gräfe und Unzer GmbH, Munich, 1979, pp. 264–265.

L-TRYPTOPHAN

Oh sleep! it is a gentle thing,
Beloved from pole to pole!
Samuel Taylor Coleridge
The Rime of the Ancient Mariner, Pt. V.

Sleep, although much sought after, is sometimes not easily achieved. That a glass of warm milk drunk before retiring is an effective remedy for mild insomnia is a truism known to all. Interestingly, this almost universal knowledge has not been given recognition in most of the standard references on pharmacy and medicine. However, in 1900, *King's American Dispensatory*[1] recorded that, "Milk is frequently of great advantage in . . . relieving *gastro-intestinal irritation, uneasiness, unrest,* and *insomnia.*" Only recently has the scientific evidence become available to support and explain this effect.

L-Tryptophan is one of the essential amino acids. That simply means it is one which the body itself cannot synthesize, and since it is essential for normal growth and development, our requirement of it must be supplied from external sources. Fortunately, it is present to the extent of 1 to 2% in most plant protein. Like many other animal proteins, casein, which makes up about 3% of cow's milk, also contains about 1.2% of L-tryptophan. The nutritional requirement of normal adult human beings approximates 500 mg. per day.[2]

Recent studies have shown that 1 gram doses of L-tryptophan reduced sleep latency (time taken to fall asleep) in both normal subjects and mild insomniacs. Doses larger than 1 gram did not produce any increased response. There is now general agreement that consumption of the compound increases subjective "sleepiness," makes one fall asleep faster, and reduces waking time.[3] As a result of these findings, and in spite of the fact that the product has not been approved for drug use, "health food" outlets, quick to recognize a potential article of commerce, began to market 100 mg. to 667 mg. tablets and capsules of the amino acid. L-Tryptophan currently averages about 30¢ for a 1 gram dose.

Advocates have pointed out that those eating a normal diet will consume 0.5 to 2 grams of the compound daily, anyway. Therefore, they view the amino acid as a food, not a drug. This view is somewhat questionable. Normally, it is consumed in relatively small amounts over extended periods of time. The probable mechanism of action of the relatively large single dose of L-tryptophan is an increase of the chemical serotonin, for which it acts as a precursor, in special nerve cells (serotoninergic neurons) of the brain.[4] While this may induce sleep, it may also induce such conditions as migraine or other forms of vascular headache which are thought to be caused by serotonin.[5]

Because no safety studies have been conducted, speculation, particularly on the safety of large doses of L-tryptophan, is probably futile. The drug is potentially useful for treating insomnia, certain kinds of pain, and even mental depression.[6,7] Whether it is completely safe is at present unknown. However, since it has been rather widely used as a sleep aid during the last several years without reports of any pronounced toxicity, its occasional use probably involves relatively little risk for normal persons.

REFERENCES

1. H. W. Felter and J. U. Lloyd: King's American Dispensatory, 18th Ed., Vol. 2. The Ohio Valley Co., Cincinnati, 1900, p. 1109.
2. The Merck Index, 7th Ed. Merck & Co., Rahway, N.J., 1960, pp. 1074–1075.
3. E. Hartmann: The Sleeping Pill. Yale University Press, New Haven, 1978, pp. 162–181.
4. V. E. Tyler, L. R. Brady, and J. E. Robbers: Pharmacognosy, 8th Ed. Lea & Febiger, Philadelphia, 1981, p. 498.
5. D. J. Dalessio: Wolff's Headache and Other Head Pain, 3rd Ed. Oxford University Press, New York, 1972, pp. 332–333.
6. C. Colvin: American Pharmacy NS19(9): 24–25, 1979.
7. J. Kingaard: Whole Foods 6(6): 18–19, 1983.

UVA URSI

If learning is a process of repetition, no one should have difficulty remembering the name of the plant which yields this drug, *Arctostaphylos uva-ursi* (L.) Spreng. and its varieties *coactylis* and *adenotricha* Fern. et Macbr. *Arctostaphylos* means bearberry in Greek, *uva ursi* means bearberry in Latin, and the plant is often called bearberry in English. But just to throw in one confusing element, it is the dried leaves, not the berries, of the widely distributed, trailing evergreen shrub of the family Ericaceae which make up its medicinal properties.[1]

In folk medicine, uva ursi is a diuretic and astringent for diseases of the bladder and kidneys. It's supposed to impart tone to the urinary passages and also to exert an antiseptic action there. This is supposed to render the drug practicable in various inflammatory diseases of the urinary tract such as urethritis, cystitis, etc.[2]

Uva ursi contains about 5% to 12% of the phenolic glycoside arbutin which hydrolyzes when taken to release hydroquinone, the principal antiseptic and astringent constituent of the plant.[3] Ursolic acid, a triterpene derivative, and isoquercetin, a flavonoid pigment, also contribute to the diuretic action.[4] Bearberry contains large amounts (15–20%) of tannin, an undesirable constituent which tends to upset the stomach. Consequently, the leaves should not be extracted with hot water, as is normally the case in preparing a tea. Rather, better to pour cold water over them and allow them to stand 12 to 24 hours before drinking. This minimizes the tannin content of the beverage.

Arbutin, or more specifically, the hydroquinone derived from it, is a pretty effective urinary antiseptic but only if taken in large doses and if the urine is alkaline. This means that consumers should avoid eating acid-rich foods, including many fruits and their juices, sauerkraut, vitamin C, and similar products.[5] Consumers must also be aware that hydroquinone, in large doses, is toxic and may cause ringing in the ears, vomiting, convulsions, and collapse. However, since the recommended dose of uva ursi is 1 gram, 3 to 6 times daily, and doses as large as 20 grams have produced no response in healthy individuals, there would seem to be minimal cause for concern.[6]

Uva ursi is an ingredient in practically all of the kidney- and bladder-type teas, large numbers of which are marketed in Europe. It appears to be a modestly effective urinary antiseptic and diuretic if properly employed. The wisdom of self-determining conditions in which it might prove helpful and then self-treating them is, of course, an individual matter.

REFERENCES

1. V. E. Tyler, L. R. Brady, and J. E. Robbers: Pharmacognosy, 8th Ed. Lea & Febiger, Philadelphia, 1981, pp. 77, 499.
2. M. Grieve: A Modern Herbal, Vol. 1. Dover Publications, New York, 1971, pp. 89–90.
3. A. Y. Leung: Encyclopedia of Common Natural Ingredients Used in Food, Drugs, and Cosmetics. John Wiley & Sons, New York, 1980, pp. 316–317.
4. D. G. Spoerke, Jr.: Herbal Medications. Woodbridge Press Publishing Co., Santa Barbara, Calif., 1980, pp. 30–31.
5. M. Pahlow: Das grosse Buch der Heilpflanzen. Gräfe und Unzer GmbH, Munich, 1979, pp. 66–70.
6. T. Sollmann: A Manual of Pharmacology, 7th Ed. W. B. Saunders, Philadelphia, 1948, p. 576.

VALERIAN

Valerian and its extracts are contained singly and in combination in literally scores of drugs and teas that are currently available on the European market. Consisting of the dried rhizome and roots (underground parts) of *Valeriana officinalis* L. of the family Valerianaceae, the drug continues to be used after more than 1000 years as a valued tranquilizer and calmative in cases of nervousness and hysteria. Other species of *Valeriana*, especially *V. mexicana* DC., contain active principles and are similarly utilized.[1]

The valerian or garden heliotrope is a tall perennial herb whose hollow stem bears opposite leaves and white or reddish flowers. It has a vertical rhizome with numerous attached rootlets which are harvested in the autumn of the second year's growth. These parts possess an extremely characteristic, disagreeable aroma arising from the contained volatile oil. The odor is said to be attractive to rats (legend has it that the Pied Piper used valerian to lure these pesky rodents from the village of Hamelin[2]).

Extensive chemical studies have been carried out recently on valerian, and a new group of active principles collectively designated as valepotriates was identified. Commercial samples of *V. officinalis* contain about 2.55% valepotriates and *V. mexicana* as much as 4.8%. An extract of the latter drug which is incorporated into a proprietary preparation sold in Germany contains 50.1% valepotriates.[3] The valepotriates are quite unstable and are deactivated by heat, mineral acids, and alkali.[4] The volatile oil contained in valerian also contributes to the sedative effect of the plant.[5] In addition, it exhibits some spasmolytic activity. By their very nature, volatile oils tend to evaporate so both of the sedative components of valerian, the valepotriates and the volatile oil, are relatively unstable ingredients. Consequently, it is easy to understand why many of the old-style pharmaceutical preparations, such as valerian tincture, or even teas made from old, improperly stored drug, would be essentially inactive.

A number of clinical studies have now shown that valerian preparations containing the active valepotriates do possess definite tranquilizing activity in small animals and in human beings.[5] There is also some sedative effect, at least in certain subjects. The incidence of undesirable side effects was found to be less than with diazepam (Valium®).[6]

Furthermore, the depressant activity was not found to be synergistic with alcohol as is the case with many synthetic tranquilizers.[7] This simply means that when valerian is taken together with alcohol, the total depressant effect is not greater than that produced by the same amount of each drug taken separately. In the case of many synthetic tranquilizers, the total effect produced when taken with alcohol is greater than if each drug were taken independently. But the synergistic effect which may cause excessive depression and even death when both tranquilizing drugs and alcohol are ingested, does not exist with the valepotriates of valerian.

It would be nice to be able to conclude the discussion of the potentially useful plant drug without including any negative statements, but this is *The New Honest Herbal*, so all aspects of the drug must be considered. The usable properties of valerian determined in the double-blind clinical trials just discussed were all carried out using standardized pharmaceutical preparations containing known amounts of active valepotriates. Would one get the same effect by drinking a tea made from the powdered drug or by taking a capsule of the same material? I doubt it.

At present, we have no assurance that the commercially purchased crude drug has any particular concentration of active ingredients. The same may be said of valerian grown in our own gardens because there is no simple procedure available to determine its potency. Until such information becomes available, and in the absence of any valepotriate-containing proprietary products (for these have not been officially evaluated for safety and efficacy and are thus not available in the United States), we can only lament the uncertainty surrounding the domestic use of this crude drug as a tranquilizer. Still, the fact that it is very widely employed and has long been popular in Europe would seem to indicate a considerable degree of practical application.

REFERENCES

1. H. W. Youngken, Textbook of Pharmacognosy, 6th Ed. The Blakiston Co., Philadelphia, 1948, pp. 852–856.
2. W. H. Hylton, Ed.: The Rodale Herb Book. Rodale Press Book Div., Emmaus, Pa., 1974, pp. 611–613.

3. F. Frosch, J. Connert, and K. Hilzinger: Deutsche Apotheker Zeitung 118: 1237–1240, 1978.
4. K.-W. von Eickstedt and S. Rahman: Arzneimittel-Forschung 19: 316–319, 1969.
5. J. Béliveau: Canadian Pharmaceutical Journal 119: 24–27, 1986.
6. W. Jansen: Therapiewoche 27: 2779–2786, 1977.
7. A. G.: Deutsche Apotheker Zeitung 121: 913, 1981.
8. K.-W. von Eickstedt: Arzneimittel-Forschung 19: 995–997, 1969.

WITCH HAZEL

A lthough only a small tree, *Hamamelis virginiana* L. is a very noticeable one, particularly in the fall. At a time when it and other trees begin to lose their leaves, witch hazel is suddenly covered with a multitude of golden yellow threadlike flowers. These often remain after the other autumn colors have disappeared, making the tree very conspicuous.

Witch hazel is a native American plant and the topical use of its leaves or bark as a poultice to reduce inflammation was apparently introduced to early settlers by the Indians.[1] Various extracts were later employed both internally and externally for their astringent properties in conditions ranging from diarrhea to hemorrhoids. Then, about the middle of the 19th century, a very different kind of witch hazel preparation was introduced. Prepared by steam distilling the dormant twigs of the plant and adding alcohol to the aromatic distillate, it was designated hamamelis water, distilled witch-hazel extract, or just plain "witch hazel." The product was intended for local application to various skin conditions; large quantities are still marketed.

Tannin is the principal active ingredient in witch hazel; the leaves contain 8%, the bark from 1% to 3%. A number of other constituents including various flavonoid pigments are also present, but whatever astringent action the drug possesses seems to be accounted for by the tannin.[2] In Europe, an alcoholic fluidextract of witch hazel is often taken internally to treat varicose veins.[3] Experiments on rabbits have shown that the drug does cause constriction of the veins, at least following injection.[4] The constituent(s) responsible for this activity remains unidentified. Interestingly enough, an alcoholic extract of the leaves was found to be much more active than an aqueous extract. Thus, anybody drinking tea prepared from the witch-hazel bark commonly sold in "health food" stores should not expect much venous-constricting effect from it.

Aside from its astringency, it is a mistake to expect much of anything in the way of useful therapeutic action from this plant. At a time when various hamamelis preparations were still listed in *The National Formulary*, one authority[5] commented, "Hamamelis is so nearly destitute of medicinal virtues that it scarcely deserves official recognition." Hamamelis leaf and the fluidextract prepared from it were dropped from the 1955 edition of the N.F.

Hamamelis water is especially interesting in that, due to its method of preparation by distillation, the final product is devoid of tannin; it is therefore essentially a mixture of 14% alcohol in water with a trace of volatile oil. The same authority just cited[5] stated that hamamelis water fulfills "the universally recognized need in American families for an embrocation [liniment] which appeals to the psychic influence of faith." Any astringent action exerted by the preparation is due to its alcohol content which approximates that of table wine. Although it is seldom applied externally, red wine at least contains some tannin, and its therapeutic value as an astringent would therefore exceed that of "witch hazel."

REFERENCES

1. J. U. Lloyd: Origin and History of all the Pharmacopeial Vegetable Drugs, Chemicals and Preparations, Vol. 1. The Caxton Press, Cincinnati, 1921, p. 162.
2. P. H. List and L. Hörhammer, Eds.: Hagers Handbuch der Pharmazeutischen Praxis, 4th Ed., Vol. 5. Springer-Verlag, Berlin, 1976, pp. 9–14.
3. P. Schauenberg and F. Paris: Guide to Medicinal Plants. Lutterworth Press, Guildford, England, 1977, pp. 291–292.
4. P. Bernard, P. Balansard, G. Balansard, and A. Bovis: Journal de Pharmacie de Belgique 27: 505–512, 1972.
5. A. Osol and G. E. Farrar, Jr., Eds.: The Dispensatory of the United States of America, 24th Ed. J. B. Lippincott, Philadelphia, 1947, pp. 528–530.

WORMWOOD

As he watered the green stuff in his glass,
and the drops fell one by one.
                    Robert Service
                    "The Shooting of Dan McGrew"

Long before the "man from the creeks" had filled Dangerous Dan McGrew full of lead while under its influence, the herb known as wormwood or absinthe had acquired a sinister reputation. Although native to Europe, this shrubby, odorous plant, *Artemesia absinthium* L. of the family Compositae, has been naturalized in the United States and occurs widely in the northeast and north central regions.[1]

As its common name wormwood implies, the herb was once used as an anthelmintic to destroy intestinal worms. Its leaves and flowering tops were also used as an aromatic bitter or tonic, a diaphoretic, and as a flavoring agent. The late Euell Gibbons recommended three different formulas for wormwood preparations, including one which would cause the user to dream of his true love.[2] For reasons I shall explain, none of these can be endorsed. Wormwood is still employed in small amounts to flavor some of the aromatic alcoholic beverages including vermouth, and to impart a fragrance to certain liniments.

Wormwood acquired its sinister reputation as a subtle poison when it became the principal flavoring ingredient in a 136-proof alcoholic beverage called absinthe. This green-colored aperitif was too strong to drink straight, so most tipplers diluted it with water as described in Service's poem. It was the "in" beverage served at all the sidewalk cafes in Paris around the turn of the century. Then, one absinthe addict, Vincent van Gogh, sliced off his own ear and mailed it to a lady friend; another, John Lanfray, murdered his pregnant wife, two daughters, and then attempted suicide while under its influence; and the impressionist, Edgar Degas, painted a truly haunting portrait of two hollow-eyed absinthe drinkers, seated at a table, oblivious to all around them as a result of the toxic beverage. Practically every civilized country in the world banned the preparation or consumption of absinthe. France, which prepared most of it and which consumed two-thirds of the world's supply, was among the last to do so, in 1915.

The principles absinthin and anabsinthin are responsible for the bitter taste of wormwood, but its pleasant aroma is due to a volatile oil which is contained in the herb in a concentration ranging between 0.25 and 1.32%. The oil, in turn, contains 3–12% of thujone (a mixture of the α- and β-forms), long believed to be the major toxic constituent in the plant.[3]

More than forty years ago the injection of thujone at levels as low as 40 mg. per kg. induced convulsions in rats, and caused fatalities when this quantity was increased to 120 mg. per kg.[4] One-half ounce of wormwood volatile oil also caused convulsions and unconsciousness in a human being, according to an ancient medical report.

Only recently have scientists been able to offer an explanation for the difference between the relatively large doses of thujone required to produce toxic effects in rats and the much smaller amounts known to impair the faculties of human beings. They propose that thujone exerts its psychotomimetic (mind-altering) effects by reacting with the same receptor sites in the brain as those which interact with THC (tetrahydrocannabinol), the active principle of marihuana.[5]

This hypothesis is supported by observing the same mind-altering effects induced by drinking absinthe and by smoking marihuana. Also, thujone and THC not only have similar molecular geometries and similar functional groups allowing them to "fit" a common receptor site without changing orientations or relative positions; they also are capable of similar types of oxidative reactions. The theory requires experimental verification, but it does explain why absinthe, even when consumed in relatively small amounts, could cause such profound mental and physical changes in habitual or even casual users.

REFERENCES

1. H. W. Youngken: Textbook of Pharmacognosy, 6th Ed. The Blakiston Co., Philadelphia, 1948, pp. 873–874.
2. E. Gibbons: Stalking the Healthful Herbs, Field Guide Ed. David McKay Co., New York, 1966, pp. 42–46.
3. H. A. Hoppe: Drogenkunde, 8th Ed., Vol. 1. Walter de Gruyter, Berlin, 1975, pp. 119–120.
4. W. L. Sampson and L. Fernandez: Journal of Pharmacology and Experimental Therapeutics 65: 275–280, 1939.
5. J. del Castillo, M. Anderson, and G. M. Rubottom: Nature 253: 365–366, 1975.

YELLOW DOCK

For hundreds of years, herbalists have been recommending the root of various species of dock for diseases of the blood and liver. These recommendations are repeated, using slightly different terminology, in modern herbal writings which describe yellow dock, Rumex crispus L. (family Polygonaceae), as a helpful alterative and laxative.[1] The term alterative refers to a drug intended for the treatment of syphilis and related venereal diseases; it is often used synonymously with "blood purifier."

Yellow dock is a perennial herb, growing up to about four feet in height, with slender leaves characterized by wavy-curled margins. This accounts for another, widely used name for the plant, curly dock. It is a native of Europe but is found growing abundantly in waste places throughout most of the United States. The deep yellow, underground parts (rhizome and roots) make up the drug, but dock greens are also eaten as a potherb. Actually, a number of closely related species are similarly employed, and when Rumex was listed in The National Formulary, R. obtusifolius L. was also designated as a source.[2]

A number of anthraquinone derivatives, including chrysophanic acid, emodin, and physcion, among others, have been identified in yellow dock.[3] These account for the drug's laxative action which is well substantiated. In fact, one study[4] showed that the total anthraquinone content of this plant's root, 2.17%, exceeded the 1.42% concentration of these principles in medicinal rhubarb (not to be confused with garden rhubarb which does not contain anthraquinones). Incidentally, rhubarb belongs to the same plant family as yellow dock; many members of the Polygonaceae contain anthraquinones accompanied by significant amounts of tannin.

It is difficult to understand how a simple laxative drug could have retained its ancient reputation for being of value in the treatment of venereal disease and its various symptoms, especially the skin conditions. This can only emphasize how uncritically the attributes, or lack of them, of various vegetable drugs are still assessed by their fans. There is absolutely no physiological or chemical evidence to support any claim of this kind of therapeutic ability for yellow dock. However, because of its content of tannin and anthraquinones, the drug's astringent and laxative properties are well established.

REFERENCES

1. M. Tierra: The Way of Herbs. Unity Press, Santa Cruz, Calif., 1980, pp. 121–122.
2. The *National Formulary*, 5th Ed. American Pharmaceutical Association, Washington, D.C., 1926, pp. 386–387.
3. P. H. List and L. Hörhammer, Eds.: Hagers Handbuch der Pharmazeutischen Praxis, 4th Ed., Vol. 6B. Springer-Verlag, Berlin, 1979, pp. 192–194.
4. J. J. Raffa Arias and C. E. Molfino: Revista Farmaceutica (Buenos Aires) 104: 151–155, 1962.

YOHIMBE

Hast du Yohimbin im Haus,
Macht der Hausfreund dir nichts aus.
Yohimbin ist grosser Mist,
Wenn's der Hausfreund selber frisst.

At first, this bit of German doggerel might seem to have little relation to a West African tree, but it is just such a plant whose bark, known as yohimbe, has long been valued as an aphrodisiac. The tree, known as *Pausinystalia yohimbe* (K. Schumann) Pierre, a member of the family Rubiaceae, is native to Cameroon, Gabon, and Congo. Its bark contains up to about 6% of a mixture of alkaloids, the principal one being yohimbine.[1]

Yohimbe and yohimbine enjoy a considerable folkloric reputation as aphrodisiacs, that is, drugs which stimulate sexual desire and performance. One recipe recommends boiling 6 to 10 teaspoonfuls of inner bark shavings in a pint of water for a few minutes, straining, sweetening, and drinking the beverage. The alkaloidal salt yohimbine hydrochloride is administered in 5 mg. doses, although there is considerable doubt as to its effectiveness in this amount. It is available as a prescription drug in a variety of combinations with other so-called sexual stimulants, including strychnine, thyroid, and methyltestosterone. Some authors recommend snuffing yohimbine to obtain both stimulant and mild hallucinogenic effects.[2]

The drug dilates the blood vessels of the skin and mucous membranes and thereby lowers blood pressure. Its alleged aphrodisiac effects are attributed not only to this enlargement of blood vessels in the sexual organs but to increased reflex excitability in the sacral (lower) region of the spinal cord. Until recently, scientific studies of the aphrodisiac properties of yohimbine had produced unimpressive results. Then, in 1984, an investigation of the effect of relatively small doses in sexually active male rats concluded that the drug definitely increased sexual arousal in the treated animals.[3] The investigators concluded that these results differed from those of earlier studies because the much larger doses of the drug previously employed produced other behavioral changes in the test animals. While it is not yet possible to draw any firm conclusions regarding the aphrodisiac effects of yohimbe and its contained alkaloids in human beings, there is certainly reason to justify further study of the herb and its use in the treatment of sexual dysfunction.[4]

Yohimbe is a monoamine oxidase inhibitor which means that tyramine-containing foods (liver, cheese, red wine, etc.) and nasal decongestants or certain diet aids containing phenylpropanolamine should be rigorously avoided if it is used. The drug also should not be taken by persons suffering from hypotension, diabetes, or from heart, liver, or kidney disease. Psychic reactions resembling anxiety have been shown to be produced by yohimbine. In the case of individuals suffering from schizophrenia, it may actually activate psychoses.[5,6] These unpleasant and potentially hazardous reactions make it impossible to recommend the use of yohimbe for self-treatment. In any event, neither it nor yohimbine is now readily available over the counter in the United States. Yohimbine is widely sold in Europe as an ingredient in a large number of preparations said to enhance sexual potency.

For those who cannot read German and are still curious, the author's English version of the introductory poem reads:

> If in the house there's yohimbine about,
> Your wife's secret lover just won't make out.
> But be careful, it may do you no good at all,
> If he finds it and takes it, then he'll have the ball.

REFERENCES

1. E. Steinegger and R. Hänsel: Lehrbuch der Pharmakognosie, 3rd Ed. Springer-Verlag, Berlin, 1972, p. 327–328.
2. L. A. Young, L. G. Young, M. M. Klein, D. M. Klein, and D. Beyer: Recreational Drugs. Collier Books, New York, 1977, pp. 207–208.
3. V. E. Tyler: Pharmacy International 7: 203–207, 1986.
4. Anon.: Lancet II: 1194–1195, 1986.
5. G. Holmberg and S. Gershon: Psychopharmacologia 2: 93–106, 1961.
6. C. G. Ingram: Clinical Pharmacology and Therapeutics 3: 345–352, 1962.

YUCCA

About 40 species of the genus *Yucca* grow in the warmer parts of North America, and a few species are hardy in colder climates. These members of the family Agavaceae are extensively cultivated, particularly in the South. The plants, with their stiff, usually sword-shaped leaves, may or may not have an erect, central stem. Many have descriptive common names which are much more widely recognized than their botanical designations. *Yucca aloifolia* L. is called Spanish-bayonet or dagger plant; *Y. brevifolia* Engelm. is the well-known Joshua tree; *Y. glauca* Nutt. ex J. Fraser is referred to as soapweed; *Y. whipplei* Torr. is Our-Lord's-candle.[1]

Yucca species, together with other agaves, are known to contain large quantities of saponins. These bitter, generally irritating principles are characterized by their capacity to foam when shaken with water. The saponins in yucca are steroid derivatives, and have been extensively studied because of their potential ability as starting materials for the synthesis of cortisone and related corticoids. The specific identity and the amounts of the numerous saponins in yucca were found to vary markedly with the part of the plant tested and the season when it was collected.[2]

The recommendation of yucca in medicine, unlike that of many plant materials we have considered, is of relatively recent origin. It stems from 1975 when the results of a study titled "Yucca Plant Saponin in the Management of Arthritis" appeared in *The Journal of Applied Nutrition*.[3] Essentially, the investigators claimed to have shown that a "saponin extract" of the "desert yucca plant," taken four times daily, was both safe and effective in treating the various forms of arthritis. Neither the species nor the plant part from which the saponin extract was obtained was revealed, nor was its method of preparation specified.

The Arthritis Foundation has analyzed the methodology and results of this study and pointed out a number of deficiencies. The investigators did not differentiate between rheumatoid arthritis and osteoarthritis, two very different diseases. Other medications, in addition to the yucca, continued to be taken by the patients. Individual dosages and lengths of treatment were very different (one week to 15 months), but results were all lumped together. Most patient response was subjective and not based on physical evidence. Some of the reported results were inconsistent.[4] Along with these objections add the unknown composition of the drug itself and the lack of assured uniformity in different lots.

Charles C. Bennett, Vice President of Public Education for the Arthritis Foundation, suggests that inquiries concerning yucca be answered ". . . by saying that there is no proper scientific evidence that yucca tablets are helpful in treating rheumatoid arthritis or osteoarthritis; that they are probably harmless; and that the real danger would be in taking yucca tablets INSTEAD OF following proper and proven treatment procedures, which could lead to irreversible joint damage and possible disabilities." Nothing need be added to this statement.

REFERENCES

1. L. H. Bailey and E. Z. Bailey: Hortus Third, Macmillan, New York, 1976, pp. 1178–1179.
2. R. Hegnauer: Chemotaxonomie der Pflanzen, Vol. 2. Birkhäuser Verlag, Basel, 1963, pp. 27–36.
3. R. Bingham, B. A. Bellew, and J. G. Bellew: Journal of Applied Nutrition 27(2–3): 45–51, 1975.
4. C. C. Bennett: Public Information Memo, The Arthritis Foundation, New York, Feb. 22, 1977.

INDEX

SUMMARIZED EVALUATION OF HERBAL REMEDIES

This chapter consists primarily of a table providing a summarized evaluation of the various herbal remedies and related products discussed in detail in each section of the previous chapter. The summary includes both the common and scientific names of the plant, the part used, the principal uses, its apparent effectiveness and probable safety.

I must add a word of caution regarding the last two categories which, in my experience, are unique inclusions in an herbal intended for popular consumption. The value judgments presented are those formed by the author after detailed study of literally thousands of books and papers devoted to natural products used as drugs. In most cases, they are not based on the outcomes of the extensive double-blind clinical studies in human beings which the Food and Drug Administration requires to *prove* a drug safe and effective. Rather, they are founded on the majority of satisfactory evidence obtained from all sources regarding each drug.

For example, in the United States, German or Hungarian chamomile has not been declared a safe and effective drug, at least as far as the FDA is concerned. The reason for this is that the FDA has not been presented with sufficient evidence to prove unequivocally its safety and efficacy as a medicinal agent. And that is because no drug company is willing to spend the money to obtain this evidence since they probably could not profit from such an investment.

Still, various types of chamomile have been used as carminative, anti-inflammatory, antispasmodic, and anti-infective agents since the time of the Egyptians. Under its Latin title Matricaria, German chamomile was granted official status first in *The United States Pharmacopeia* and then in *The National Formulary* for an extended period (108 years). This status did not end until 1950. With the exception of an infrequent allergic reaction in sensitive individuals, reports of untoward side effects from chamomile are essentially lacking in the literature. Both the crude plant material and the volatile oil obtained from it are "Generally Recognized As Safe" when used as flavoring agents for foods. In this capacity, they appear on the so-called GRAS list of the Food and Drug Administration.

Scores of medicinal chamomile products ranging from the crude drug incorporated in various medicinal tea mixtures to preparations containing the purified volatile oil are marketed in European countries. Scientific papers from those countries report favorable therapeutic results with German chamomile in both small animals and human beings. For all of these reasons, in the following table, chamomile has been rated as an apparently safe and probably effective drug, *when used appropriately.*

All the value judgments given in the table, both positive and negative, are based on similar evidence and reasoning. If used with this understanding, the table will provide the busy reader at a single glance the essential information about each drug included in this book.

Common Name	Source	Part Used	Principal Uses	Apparent Efficacy[a]	Probable Safety[a]
Alfalfa	Medicago sativa	leaves and tops	antiarthritic, lower cholesterol	–	+
Aloe	Aloe barbadensis	1. fresh juice 2. dried juice	wound healing, burns cathartic	+ +	+ +
Angelica	Angelica archangelica	root, fruit, leaves	1. antiflatulent, emmenagogue, etc. 2. flavor	– +	– +
Apricot Pits (Laetrile)	Prunus armeniaca	seed kernels	anticancer	–	–
Arnica	Arnica spp.	flower heads	anti-inflammatory analgesic	+	+
Barberry	Mahonia or Berberis spp.	rhizome and roots	antibacterial, astringent	+	+
Bayberry	Myrica cerifera	1. root bark 2. berries	astringent (diarrhea) fragrant wax candles	+ +	±[b] +
Betony	Stachys officinalis	leaves and tops	astringent (diarrhea, sore throat)	+	±[b]
Black Cohosh	Cimicifuga racemosa	rhizome and roots	antirheumatic, uterine problems, etc.	–	±
Blue Cohosh	Caulophyllum thalictroides	rhizome and roots	uterine stimulant, emmenagogue, etc.	+	–
Boneset	Eupatorium perfoliatum	leaves and tops	1. break up colds and flu 2. induce sweating	– +	+ +
Borage	Borago officinalis	leaves and tops	diuretic, astringent (diarrhea)	– to ±	±
Bran	Triticum aestivum	outer seed coat	Increase dietary fiber, benefit various gastrointestinal conditions	+	+
Broom	Cytisus scoparius	flowering tops	mind-altering properties (smoked)	+	–
Buchu	Barosma spp.	leaves	urinary antiseptic, diuretic	± to +	+
Burdock	Arctium spp.	root	alterative, treatment of skin disorder	–	+
Butcher's-Broom	Ruscus aculeatus	rhizome and root	improve circulation	±	+

Common Name	Source	Part Used	Principal Uses	Apparent Efficacy[a]	Probable Safety[a]
Caffeine-Containing Plants					
Coffee	Coffea arabica	seeds	} central stimulant	+	±
Tea	Camellia sinensis	leaves and leaf buds			
Kola	Cola nitida	cotyledons (seed leaves)			
Cacao	Theobroma cacao	seeds			
Guarana	Paullinia cupana	seeds			
Mate	Ilex paraguariensis	leaves			
Calamus	Acorus calamus	rhizome	febrifuge, digestive aid	±	– or +
Calendula (Marigold)	Calendula officinalis	ligulate florets (flower parts)	facilitate wound healing	–	+
Canaigre	Rumex hymenosepalus	root	tonic	–	–[b]
Capsicum	Capsicum spp.	fruits	rubifacient; stomachic	+	+
Catnip	Nepeta cataria	leaves and tops	1. digestive acid, sleep-aid	±	+
			2. mind-altering properties (smoked)	–	±
Chamomiles and Yarrow	Matricaria chamomilla, Anthemis nobilis, Achillea millefolium	flower heads, flower heads, flowering herb	carminative, anti-inflammatory, antispasmodic, anti-infective	+	+
Chaparral	Larrea tridentata	leaves and twigs	alterative, anticancer	–	–
Chickweed	Stellaria media	leaves and stems	treatment of skin disorders, various internal ailments	–	+
Chicory	Chicorium intybus	root	caffeine-free beverage	+	+
Coltsfoot	Tussilago farfara	leaves and/or flower heads	antitussive (coughs), demulcent	+	–
Comfrey	Symphytum officinale	rhizome and roots, leaves	general healing agent	+	–

Common Name	Latin Name	Plant Part	Use		
Cucurbita	Curcurbita spp.	seeds	teniagfuge (expel intestinal worms)	+	+
Damiana	Turnera diffusa var. aphrodisiaca	leaves	aphrodisiac	−	+
Dandelion	Taraxacum officinale	1. rhizome and roots 2. leaves	digestive aid, laxative, diuretic	± ±	+ +
Devil's Claw	Harpagophytum procumbuns	secondary storage roots	antirheumatic	−	+
Dong Quai	Angelica polymorpha var. sinensis	root	uterine tonic, antispasmodic, alterative	±	−
Echinacea	Echinacea angustifolia	rhizome and roots	anti-infective, wound healing	+	+
Evening Primrose	Oenothera biennis	seed oil	treatment of atopic eczema; mastalgia	+	+
Eyebright	Euphrasia officinalis	entire overground plant	treatment of eye diseases (conjunctivitis)	−	−
Fennel	Foeniculum vulgare	fruits (seeds)	stomachic, carminative	+	+
Fenugreek	Trigonella foenumgraecum	seeds	1. demulcent, stomachic 2. flavor	± ±	+ +
Feverfew	Chrysanthemum parthenium	leaves	migraine preventive	+	+
Fo-Ti	Polygonum multiflorum	tuberous root	1. cathartic 2. rejuvenation	+ −	,+ +
Garlic and Other Alliums	Allium sativum (garlic) Allium cepa (onion) Allium ampeloprasum (leek) Allium ascalonicum (scallion)	bulbs and occasionally leaves	treatment of atherosclerosis and high blood pressure, gastrointestinal ailments	+	+
Gentian	Gentiana lutea	rhizome and roots	appetite stimulant, digestive aid	+	+
Ginger	Zingiber officinale	rhizome	motion sickness preventive	+	+

Common Name	Source	Part Used	Principal Uses	Apparent Efficacy[a]	Probable Safety[a]
Ginseng and Related Drugs	Panax pseudoginseng (Oriental ginseng) Panax quinquefolius (American ginseng) Panax notoginseng (Tienchi-ginseng) Acanthopanax senticosus (Siberian ginseng)	roots	Adaptogen, tonic, cure-all antistress agent	±	±
Goldenseal	Hydrastis canadensis	rhizome and roots	bitter tonic, digestive aid, treatment of genitourinary disorders	± to +	+
Gotu Kola	Centella asiatica	leaves	promote longevity, aphrodisiac	–	±
Hawthorn	Crataegus oxycantha	fruits (haws), leaves, flowers	dilate blood vessels, lower blood pressure	+	+
Hibiscus	Hibiscus sabdariffa	flowers	laxative, diuretic	± to +	+
Honey	Apis mellifera	saccharine secretion	1. antiarthritic, sedative 2. nutrient, sweetener	– / +	+ / +
Hops	Humulus lupulus	fruits (strobiles)	1. sedative, sleep aid 2. mind-altering action	± to + / ±	+ / ±
Horehound	Marrubium vulgare	leaves and tops	expectorant (coughs)	+	+
Horsetail	Equisetum arvense	overground plant	diuretic and astringent in kidney and bladder ailments	– to ±	+
Hydrangea	Hydrangea arborescens	rhizome and roots	diuretic and treatment of kidney stones	–	±
	Hydrangea paniculata	leaves	mind-altering action (smoked)	+	–
Hyssop	Hyssopus officinalis	leaves	expectorant (coughs and colds)	+	+
Jojoba Oil	Simmondsia chinensis	expressed from seeds	1. antisebum shampoos 2. emollient lotions, cosmetics	± / +	+ / +

Common Name	Scientific Name	Plant Part	Action/Use		
Juniper	Juniperus communis	fruits (berries)	diuretic	+	±
Kelp	Laminaria, Macrocystis Nereocystis, and Fucus spp.	entire plant	1. bulk laxative, demulcent 2. control obesity, atherosclerosis	+ -	+ +
Lettuce Opium	Lactuca virosa and related species	dried latex	1. sedative, analgesic 2. mind-altering action (smoked)	- -	+ ±
Licorice	Glycyrrhiza glabra	rhizome and roots	expectorant, demulcent, flavor	+	+ to -
Life Root	Senecio aureus	entire plant	emmenagogue, treatment of uterine diseases	±	-
Linden Flowers	Tilia spp.	flowers	diaphoretic, beverage	+	+
Lobelia	Lobelia inflata	leaves and tops	1. nauseant expectorant 2. mind-altering action	+ +	± -
Lovage	Levisticum officinale	1. rhizome and roots 2. leaves	diuretic, carminative flavor	+ +	+ +
Mistletoe	Phoradendron tomentosum subsp. macrophyllum (American mistletoe)	leaves	stimulate smooth muscle, increase blood pressure	±	-
	Viscum album and subsp. (European mistletoe)	leaves	antispasmodic, reduce blood pressure	±	-
Mormon Tea	Ephedra nevadensis	stems	1. alterative, tonic 2. diuretic, astringent (diarrhea)	- +	±[b] ±[b]
Muira Puama	Ptychopetalum olacoides and P. uncinatum	stem-wood, root	aphrodisiac	-	±
Mullein	Verbascum thapsus	leaves, flowers	demulcent, emollient, astringent	+	+
Myrrh	Commiphora spp.	oleo-gum-resin	astringent, protective, fragrance	+	+
Nettle	Urtica dioica	overground plant	1. diuretic 2. antiasthmatic, antirheumatic, stimulate hair growth	+ -	+ +

Common Name	Source	Part Used	Principal Uses	Apparent Efficacy[a]	Probable Safety[a]
New Zealand Green-Lipped Mussel	Perna canaliculus	entire organism	antiarthritic	−	+
Pangamic Acid	Prunus armeniaca or synthetic	chemical or chemical mixture	various, detoxify poisonous products in human system	−	− to ±
Papaya	Carica papaya	1. dried latex 2. leaves	digestive aid, vermifuge	−	+
Parsley	Petroselinum crispum	1. leaves and stems 2. fruit (seeds)	digestive aid, diuretic digestive aid, diuretic, emmenagogue	± +	+ ± to +
Passion Flower	Passiflora incarnata	flowering and fruiting top	sedative, calmative	± to +	+
Pau d'Arco	Tabebuia spp.	bark	anticancer	−	±
Pennyroyal	Hedeoma pulegioides (American pennyroyal) Mentha pulegium (European pennyroyal)	leaves oil	carminative, diaphoretic, emmenagogue emmenagogue, abortifacient	± + to ±	+ −
Peppermint	Mentha piperita	leaves	stomachic, carminative, flavor	+	+
Poke Root	Phytolacca americana	root	alterative, antirheumatic, anticancer, cathartic, etc.	−	−
Pollen	seed-bearing plants	microspores (male reproductive elements)	tonic, treatment of various debilitating conditions	−	− to ±
Propolis	bee hives – originally from conifer and poplar trees	resinous material	antibacterial activity (tuberculosis), gastrointestinal disturbances	±	+
Raspberry	Rubus idaeus	leaves	astringent, stimulant	+	+[b]
Red Bush Tea	Aspalathus linearis	leaves and fine twigs	refreshing beverage	+	+

Common Name	Scientific Name	Part	Uses		
Red Clover	*Trifolium pratense*	flowers	alterative, anticancer treatment	–	+
Rose Hips	*Rosa* spp.	fruits	antiscorbutic	+	+
Rosemary	*Rosmarinus officinalis*	leaves and/or tops	tonic, diaphoretic, stomachic, spice, flavor	+	+
Royal Jelly	*Apis mellifera*	pharyngeal gland secretion	tonic, prevent aging	–	+
Rue	*Ruta graveolens*	leaves	antispasmodic, emmenagogue	+	– to ±
Sage	*Salvia officinalis*	leaves	1. astringent, anhidrotic (reduce secretions)	+	– to ±
			2. flavor	+	+
St. John's Wort	*Hypericum perforatum*	leaves and tops	tranquilizer, anti-inflammatory	+	+
Sarsaparilla	*Smilax* spp.	roots	1. alterative	–	+
			2. diuretic, flavor	+	+
Sassafras	*Sassafras albidum*	root bark	1. stimulant, antispasmodic, sudorific, antirheumatic, tonic	–	–
			2. flavor	+	–
Savory	*Satureja hortensis* (summer savory)	overground plant	1. carminative, appetite stimulant, antidiarrhea	+	+
Savory	*Satureja montana* (winter savory)	overground plant	2. aphrodisiac	–	+
			decrease sex drive	–	+
Saw Palmetto	*Serenoa repens*	ripe fruits	1. diuretic, treatment of cystitis and prostatitis	±	+
			2. increase size of mammary glands; stimulate sexual vigor	–	+
Schisandra	*Schisandra chinensis*	fruits	stimulant; liver protectant	±	±
Scullcap	*Scutellaria lateriflora*	overground plant	tonic, tranquilizing effects, antispasmodic	–	+
Senaga Snakeroot	*Polygala senega*	root	expectorant, diaphoretic, emetic	+	+

Common Name	Source	Part Used	Principal Uses	Apparent Efficacy[a]	Probable Safety[a]
Senna	Cassia acutifolia (Alexandria senna) Cassia angustifolia (Tinnevelly senna)	leaflets	cathartic	+	+
Spirulina	Spirulina spp. (blue-green algae)	entire plants	1. nutrient 2. appetite supressant	+ − to ±	+ +
Tansy	Chrysanthemum vulgare	leaves and tops	anthelmintic, tonic, emmenagogue	±	− to ±
L-Tryptophan	Casein	amino acid	sleep aid, antidepressant	+	+
Uva Ursi	Arctostaphylos uva-ursi	leaves	diuretic, urinary antiseptic, astringent	+	+
Valerian	Valerian officinalis Valerian mexicana	rhizome and roots	tranquilizer, calmative	+	+
Witch Hazel	Hamamelis virginiana	leaves, bark	astringent	+	+
Wormwood	Artemesia absinthium	leaves and tops	anthelmintic, tonic, mind-altering action, flavor	+	−
Yellow Dock	Rumex crispus	rhizome and roots	astringent, laxative	+	+[b]
Yohimbe	Pausinystalia yohimbe	bark	aphrodisiac, sexual stimulant	+	±
Yucca	Yucca spp.	leaves	antiarthritic	−	+

1 The table does not comment on the desirability or feasibility of using any of these remedies, even those indicated as being apparently efficacious and probably safe. The interested reader should consult the text for detailed explanations of the many complex factors regarding the use of these drugs which could not be included in this brief summary.

+ = Effective, safe in normal individuals.

± = Efficacy or safety inconclusive.

− = Ineffective, not safe.

a = When used appropriately. See specific monograph for details of administration.

b = All tannin-rich drugs may have carcinogenic potential in long-term usage.